The Vaccinators

The Vaccinators

SMALLPOX, MEDICAL
KNOWLEDGE, AND THE
"OPENING" OF JAPAN

Ann Jannetta

STANFORD UNIVERSITY PRESS
STANFORD, CALIFORNIA

Stanford University Press
Stanford, California

The Japan Iron and Steel Federation Endowment Fund of the University of Pittsburgh provided a subvention to support the publication of this book

Printed in the United States of America on acid-free, archival-quality paper

Library of Congress Cataloging-in-Publication Data
Jannetta, Ann Bowman, 1932-
  The vaccinators : smallpox, medical knowledge, and the 'opening' of Japan / Ann Jannetta.
    p. ; cm.
  Includes bibliographical references and index.
  ISBN 978-0-8047-5489-7 (cloth : alk. paper)
  ISBN 978-0-8047-8690-4 (pbk. : alk. paper)
  1. Smallpox—Vaccination—Japan—History. 2. Smallpox vaccine—Japan—History. 3.
Smallpox—Japan—History. I. Title.
  [DNLM: 1. Smallpox Vaccine—history—Japan. 2. Diffusion of Innovation—Japan. 3.
History, 19th Century—Japan. 4. Smallpox—history—Japan. 5. Social Change—history—
Japan. WC 588 J34v 2007]
  RC183.7.J3J36 2007
  614.5'210952—dc22

                                                      2006035450

Typeset by inari in 11/14 Adobe Garamond

For Evelyn and Thomas Rawski

Contents

Illustrations

Tables

Conventions Used

· Chinese and Japanese names in the text, notes, and references follow the Japanese convention: surname followed by personal name, except when an author has published in English and chosen the Western order for his or her name. Japanese men were commonly known by more than one name. In this case, an alternative name is provided in brackets.

· Dates in the text are given according to the Western (Gregorian) calendar. When a Japanese date is required for a Japanese source, the pre-1872 Japanese calendar date is also given in parentheses or in a note.

· Chinese characters (*kanji*) for Japanese book titles and the names of institutions discussed in the text are provided in the glossary.

· The names of Chinese authors and book titles use pinyin transliteration except when the author and title are commonly cited using a Wade-Giles transliteration.

Preface

The Vaccinators is a book about connections. It analyzes the accelerated expansion of networks of knowledge across time and space by tracking the transmission of a new and revolutionary medical technology from its origins in rural England to the Japanese Islands in the first half of the nineteenth century. This new technology, "vaccination," used a live virus taken from cows infected with cowpox to immunize children against smallpox; once it became known that vaccination actually worked, a demand for cowpox vaccine developed quickly. Meeting this sudden demand was no simple matter. The global distribution of cowpox was limited, and even in places where the disease could be found, it was not always prevalent. This meant that distributing live cowpox virus required transporting it from Europe to the rest of the world, and soon it became clear that the virus did not travel well. Hence, the global transmission of cowpox vaccine and vaccination would rely upon a human network that could distribute the vaccine while maintaining the vitality of the fragile virus.

Why vaccination? My original interest in smallpox and vaccination goes back half a century, to August 1953, when I found myself in the Amsterdam airport without the required documents to return home. At that time, smallpox was still a devastating disease in many parts of the world, and no one was permitted to enter the United States without a valid vaccination certificate. I had been vaccinated before leaving for Europe two months earlier; however, while traveling in Italy I had contracted polio, and I was returning home unexpectedly and without my vaccination papers. Large international airports had medical staff on hand to perform routine immunizations, and persons traveling without vaccination certificates were vaccinated on the spot. So, with a minimum of fuss, I was vaccinated in the Amsterdam airport during a short layover. I attribute my long-standing interest in disease transmission, and the diffusion of medical knowledge to thwart that transmission, to that experience.

There are other reasons to examine the social history of vaccination. First and foremost, it provides an excellent example of how human ingenuity and international cooperation eradicated a universal disease that had been afflicting human societies for centuries. Such ingenuity and cooperation are still needed. National governments are presently considering the possibility that the known stores of smallpox virus, allegedly imprisoned in high-security freezers in the United States and Russia, might fall into the hands of terrorists who could unleash the virus into a global population whose immunity, acquired over two centuries of public health measures based on vaccination, has been lost. Today public health officials are trying to prepare for just such a catastrophe without alarming a public that has been spared the ravages of smallpox. Second, holding in check new diseases that now threaten the global community requires the same ingenuity and international cooperation.

The social history of vaccination and the eradication of smallpox is a transnational history that connects many national histories. My intent here is to analyze the impact of a new foreign medical technology on Japan during the last-half century of Tokugawa rule. In *Epidemics and Mortality in Early Modern Japan*, I argue that before the opening of Japan's ports in 1859, a *cordon sanitaire* protected Japan from some of the most important diseases of the early modern world. Using contemporaneous accounts of epidemics and demographic records, I was able to demonstrate the absence of diseases that were common elsewhere, and to conclude that certain diseases failed to reach premodern Japan. The reasons, I believe, were Japan's protected geographical position beyond the major world trade routes, and the xenophobic policies of Japan's Tokugawa rulers. My research for *The Vaccinators* reinforces this belief: for thirty years, deliberate efforts to export cowpox virus to Japan failed. The book examines the reasons for this failure, explores the consequences of Japan's self-imposed seclusion policies which contributed to this failure, and considers the role of Western medical knowledge in "opening" Japan to international influences before the arrival of Western gun boats in the 1850s.

* * *

The ideas in this book developed over many years, and I would like to acknowledge the contributions and help of many individuals. I first wish to acknowledge the assistance provided by various entities at the University of Pittsburgh: the Department of History, the Japan Faculty Council, the Asian Studies Center, the Japan Iron and Steel Federation Endowment, the Hewlitt International Faculty Grant Program, and the Faculty of Arts and Sciences Summer Grant Program. I have received funding to support research trips to Japan, the Netherlands, and the United Kingdom, as well as release time from teaching to work on this project. I also wish to recognize the contributions of the expert staff at the University's East Asian Library—Hiroyuki Good, Sachie Noguchi, Agnes Wen, and Haihui Zhang—all of whom helped me at various stages; and William Johnston and Alec Sarkas who prepared the illustrations for publication. Special thanks go to Valerie Hansen of Yale University and Richard Rubinger at Indiana University, who read the entire manuscript and offered important insights and recommendations for improving it.

Colleagues and institutional support in Japan made my research on this book possible. A Japan Foundation Research Grant in 1992–1993 allowed me to spend a year in Japan to investigate pertinent Japanese sources. My sponsor and mentor during that fellowship year was Professor Sakai Shizu, M.D., whose knowledge of my subject and whose helpful staff at Juntendō's Medical History Department proved invaluable. Professor Satō Kiyoshi, M.D., Professor and Chairman, Department of Neurosurgery and presently General Director of the Juntendō University Medical Institute, generously made his hospital office space available to me. Drs. Fukase Yasuaki, M.D., Kimura Sentarō, M.D., and the late Soekawa Masao, D.V.M., at the Kitasato Institute, helped me find and interpret Japanese sources relevant to the introduction of vaccination.

Dr. Takagi Kiyoko worked with me on daunting translation problems, and Mrs. Miyatake Yasuko, my expert research assistant, has become a valued friend. I wish also to acknowledge the many kindnesses of the house staff at The International House of Japan, which I regard as my second home; and the help of the I-House Library staff, which is famous for directing scholars to even the most obscure sources.

Colleagues at Leiden University, Professors Harm Beukers, Leonard Blussé, and Peter Boomgaard, and the graduate students and staff at the Institute for the History of European Expansion, made my research in the Netherlands both possible and pleasant. Frans-Paul van der Putten, an exceptionally talented researcher, was my guide to the Dutch archival sources at The

Hague, and the translator of the Dutch and German language sources cited and quoted in this book. His interest in the issues which I was pursuing made our collaboration an especially enjoyable one. Martha Chaiklin and Cynthia Viallé were also especially helpful. I have not ever had a more profitable research experience in a country where I neither speak nor read the language.

Among those closer to home, I wish to thank the library staff at the Academy of Medicine in New York City, whose help finding rare nineteenth-century European medical books made it possible to determine the origins of the books translated by Japanese physicians.

I also acknowledge the encouragement and assistance of colleagues and friends, all of whom heard far more about smallpox and vaccination than they could possibly have wanted to know. They include Margaret Forbes, Karen Gerhard, Naoko Gunji, Helen Hopper, Liu Shi-yung, Elizabeth Mertz, Geoffrey Parker, Linda Penkower, Christopher Piehler, J. Thomas Rimer, Carolyn Schumacher, Richard Smethurst, James and Rubie Watson, and Junko Yamamoto. I am indebted to Muriel Bell, senior editor at Stanford University Press, and Judith Hibbard for their professional support in producing this book. I am solely responsible for the errors and flaws that remain.

Finally, my debt to Evelyn and Thomas Rawski, whose helpful advice and long-standing interest in this book have been unstinting, is far greater than I can say. I dedicate this book to them.

Introduction

In March 1854, when Commodore Matthew C. Perry of the United States Navy sailed into Edo Bay with a squadron of five ships to demand a commercial treaty with Japan's Tokugawa shogunate, he knew he had done something remarkable. From the standpoint of Western nations in search of new markets, Japan was a "closed" country. Although challenged, this view remains largely intact today. At symposia and workshops held in 2004 on the 150th anniversary of Commodore Perry's "opening" of Japan, scholars debated the significance of complex issues related to Perry's arrival in Japan, and historians still question just how closed or open Japan really was in the final decades of Tokugawa rule.

Until 1868, Japan was ruled by the Tokugawa house, a military family that had established a government in the town of Edo in northeastern Japan in 1600. This government, called the Tokugawa or Edo *bakufu,* was headed by a series of hereditary shogun, fifteen in all, which remained in power for two and a half centuries. Tokugawa Japan was divided into approximately 250 domains: one-fourth of these domains were ruled directly by the

Tokugawa *bakufu,* and three-fourths were ruled by military overlords who had pledged fealty to the Tokugawa house. By 1725, Edo had become the largest city in the world; Kyoto remained the residence of the Japanese Emperor and the formal capital of Japan; and Osaka, on the Inland Sea, developed into a large merchant city. Nagasaki, on the southern island of Kyushu, was the only port permitted to conduct foreign trade. These cities were administered directly by a commissioner appointed by the Tokugawa *bakufu.*

To Western seafaring nations aggressively expanding their mercantile activities into the North Pacific, Japan's refusal to open its ports to foreign ships was extremely irritating. More than two centuries earlier, the Tokugawa shoguns—Japan's military rulers after 1600—closed Japan's ports by government edict in an attempt to limit contact between the Japanese and foreign nationals. The exception was the port of Nagasaki, where Chinese and Dutch merchants were authorized to conduct foreign trade at two tiny trading posts in Nagasaki Bay. Other foreign nationals were forbidden to enter Japan on pain of death, and Japanese nationals were forbidden to leave Japan and then return. Over the next two centuries, ingenious ways were devised to circumvent these directives; but, for the most part, the anti-foreign policies of the Tokugawa government were still firmly in place and operating effectively as late as 1850.

The Vaccinators examines Japan's less dramatic "opening" to Western medical knowledge in the half-century before Perry's arrival. It argues that Japanese physicians who were receptive to this knowledge strongly influenced the direction an "open" Japan would take. It focuses on the strategies of Japanese physicians who, in collaboration with Dutch merchants and influential Japanese patrons, forged a national network in support of Jennerian vaccination, a Western technology to prevent smallpox—Japan's most devastating disease. Japan's physicians used the promise of vaccination to forge lasting social and political alliances, professional networks, and public health institutions. They were a catalyst for Japan's rapid and successful modernization a century later.

Why physicians? Japanese physicians were one of the few occupational groups in Tokugawa society with the freedom to look for practical solutions outside Japan. Japan's medical tradition had always relied heavily on foreign sources. Chinese medicine held a place of honor in Japan for centuries, and during the Tokugawa period Chinese-style medicine was the orthodoxy taught in the Tokugawa Medical College and in the schools of Japan's numerous domains as well. Chinese medical books and medicines were imported regularly from China. In the sixteenth century, Western medical techniques, especially surgery, which was not practiced in China, attracted the most attention in Japan, especially in and around Nagasaki where Western influences were strongest.

In theory, medical knowledge is apolitical. Useful knowledge that can save lives and improve the quality of life can often circumvent political divisions, and political leaders of all sorts may actively seek such knowledge. In the late eighteenth century, a few Edo physicians became interested in Western anatomy books that Dutch merchants had brought to Japan. These men were known as *rangaku,* or Dutch learning, scholars. They could understand the anatomy books, in part, through drawings of the human body, and soon recognized that the drawings in Western books differed markedly from those in Chinese medical books. This discovery spurred greater interest in Western medicine and a realization that the ability to read Dutch would enhance one's comprehension of the Western medical and scientific texts that were being brought to Japan with increasing frequency.

During the late eighteenth century, *rangaku* scholars, most of whom were physicians, became the major repository of knowledge about the West. Many *rangaku* scholars were retainers of the Tokugawa *bakufu,* while others were retainers of *daimyō,* regional lords who also maintained permanent residences in Edo. Their official function as retainers was to stay informed about useful foreign medical knowledge. Sources of such knowledge were extremely limited, however—limited to medical books randomly brought to Japan by the Dutch and Chinese, and occasional conversations with Dutch merchants who came to Edo each year to pay their respects to the shogun. Even so, by the nineteenth century, *rangaku* scholars were energetically engaged in consulting both of these sources.

Physicians who practiced Western-style medicine were called *ranpō* (Dutch-method) physicians. In the early nineteenth century, both *rangaku* scholars and *ranpō* physicians began to form social and intellectual connections and to gain influence in Edo. While the distinction between *rangaku* scholars and *ranpō* physicians is not always clear cut, it is analytically useful to distinguish between those who were predominantly scholars and those who were medical practitioners. The term *ranpō* physician is used here to refer to private, practicing physicians who treated patients and taught students for a fee, as opposed to *rangaku* scholars who held an office and were paid a stipend. However, unlike most other Japanese at this time, physicians were relatively free to study and practice medicine as they saw fit. As long as they avoided offering critical political opinions, they could study what and where they wished with little interference.

The Vaccinators tracks the global transmission of Jennerian vaccination from its origins in rural England to Japan half a century later. The available sources for studying this transmission are abundant because the process of procuring the necessary vaccine produced a remarkable paper trail: personal letters, government reports, requests for vaccine, ships' logs, and so on. These sources reveal the structure of human and institutional connections that underlay the global diffusion of a medical technology that had the potential to save millions of lives. A widespread understanding of the promise of vaccination rapidly created a global demand for the precious vaccine. And this demand, in turn, forged personal relationships between physicians and patients, churches and parishioners; diplomatic relationships between allies and foes; commercial relationships between trading partners; and power relationships between colonizers and colonized.

The effective control of any infectious disease has three main requirements:

1. The sharing of knowledge, resources, and personnel among individuals and nations.
2. The collection, storing, and accessibility of evidence demonstrating both success and failure.
3. Recognition of the public's health as an element of national power, and the development of institutions to control disease and lower mortality rates.

Few societies could meet all of these requirements at the beginning of the nineteenth century. However, by the end of the century, several countries, including Japan, were meeting many of them.

The open borders that enabled European physicians and surgeons to study medicine at universities, and to serve in armies and hospitals throughout Europe, meant that the exchange of medical information was an integral part of medical education. French Huguenots studied in Edinburgh, and German nationals studied in the Netherlands. Publishing played a major role in disseminating information across political boundaries: medical texts and journals were widely read and quickly translated into both Latin and the vernacular European languages, and medical and scientific societies provided a forum where physicians could present their findings and debate theoretical and practical issues related to the practice of medicine. This intra-European cross-fertilization produced a medical culture that encouraged experimentation and the sharing of information, a culture that later was exported to the colonies of the various European nation-states.

The institutions that supported this Western medical culture were entirely absent in Japan. There were no universities or medical societies, and the Tokagawa *bakufu* regarded groups that assembled to discuss common problems as a threat. There were no medical journals, and most medical treatises remained in manuscript form and were circulated privately. The sons of the *daimyō* retainers were eligible to study medicine at domain schools, but medical training normally was acquired by attending a private medical school, or *juku,* or by taking an apprenticeship with a medical practitioner. Although this does not signify the absence of a strong medical tradition in Japan, there were no academic medical institutions, in the European sense, to connect physicians from different parts of Japan. Medical knowledge was transmitted vertically through hereditary medical lineages that were inclined to guard their secrets jealously. The transmission of medical knowledge in Japan was almost entirely a private matter.

Smallpox, on the other hand, was a public matter. Smallpox was everyman's disease, and its eradication required a public health mentality—access to professional expertise, the exercise of governmental authority, coordination between multiple jurisdictions, good record keeping, and the support of the public, all of which required sharing medical knowledge and open access to information within society. In Japan the defeat of smallpox required a social transformation. To a large extent, this transformation was well underway by the end of the nineteenth century. Social networks had been transformed into universities, publishing houses, professional societies, and a new government bureaucracy attuned to the importance of the public's health.

The advent of this transformation can be seen in the early decades of the nineteenth century by analyzing the activities of Japan's vaccinators, *ranpō* physicians who acted on foreign medical knowledge to alleviate the centuries-old problem of smallpox.

Chapter 1, "Confronting Smallpox," introduces the universal problem of smallpox in early modern societies. It reviews methods of combatting this devastating disease before 1800, focusing on an "Eastern innovation," a technique known as "variolation," knowledge of which spread from East to West in the seventeenth and eighteenth centuries. Variolation used live smallpox virus to immunize children against smallpox, but fighting smallpox with smallpox was a dangerous business. Hence, the discovery of an alternative method by Edward Jenner at the end of the eighteenth century revolutionized medical thinking and mobilized advocates, and opponents, everywhere.

Chapter 2, "Jenner's Cowpox Vaccine," considers the social, political, and institutional frameworks within which Edward Jenner conceived and presented his hypothesis to a receptive world—that cowpox virus, *Variolae vaccinae,* could be used to prevent smallpox. This chapter demonstrates the vital importance of transnational networks in the early transmission of vaccination, which would prove to be a revolutionary new medical technology. The global diffusion of *V. vaccinae* relied on loosely connected, often personal networks that could respond quickly to different circumstances. In less than a decade, a human web—seamen, diplomats, soldiers, merchants, officials, doctors, scientists—had transmitted the virus virtually everywhere in the world. The most notable exception was Japan, where *V. vaccinae* would not penetrate Japan's *cordon sanitaire* for another half-century. The remaining chapters analyze the reasons for this delay and for the remarkable reception that attended the arrival of vaccination in Japan at mid-century.

Chapter 3, "Engaging the Periphery," examines the circumstances in which knowledge of vaccination reached Japan at the beginning of the nineteenth century. It introduces the writings of Baba Sajūrō, a young and talented Dutch interpreter, whose unusual linguistic abilities enabled him to interact with foreigners who spoke Dutch, Russian, French, and English. Baba Sajūrō would be the first person to write about vaccination in Japanese. This chapter concludes that internal, structural barriers, not Japan's foreign policy *per se,* prevented the movement of useful knowledge from Japan's periphery to the Tokugawa shogun's government in Edo.

Chapter 4, "The Dutch Connection: Batavia, Nagasaki, and Edo," examines the ways in which internal barriers to foreign knowledge began to fall in the early decades of the nineteenth century. The Napoleonic Wars stranded the Dutch merchants stationed on Dejima in Nagasaki for many years, a circumstance that permitted much greater interaction between the Dutch and Japanese than previously had been possible—interactions that had long-term consequences. This chapter documents numerous attempts by the Dutch to export cowpox vaccine from the Dutch East Indies to Japan, and shows the close collaboration that developed between Japan's *ranpō* physicians and the

Dutch factory personnel. It demonstrates the importance of the Dutch presence in Japan as a catalyst in the opening of Japan to Western knowledge.

Chapter 5, "Constructing a Network: The *Ranpō* Physicians," introduces seven practitioners of Western-style medicine who became staunch advocates of vaccination before cowpox vaccine became available. These men were newcomers to medicine who relied on strong social networks—teacher-student bonds, marriage and adoption alliances, and the support of powerful patrons —to build successful careers in Western-style medicine. Adopting Jennerian vaccination as their *cause célèbre*, they created a national network of activists open to foreign ideas.

Chapter 6, "The Vaccinators," tracks the rapid transmission of cowpox vaccine throughout the Japanese Islands in the summer and fall of 1849. A detailed chronology shows how *ranpō* physicians employed the social networks they had created over a period of thirty years to distribute cowpox vaccine, to educate physicians about how to use it, and, within six months, to establish private vaccination clinics throughout the archipelago. The speed and extent of this transmission reveal the national scale of Japan's vaccination network.

Chapter 7, "Engaging the Center," analyzes the ways in which Japan's vaccinators finally engaged the Tokugawa *bakufu* in their efforts to promote vaccination in the city of Edo. With the opening of the Otamagaike Vaccination Clinic in Edo in 1858, the sponsors of the Clinic and their descendents established themselves as the founding generation of modern medicine and public health in Japan. The private initiatives of Japan's *ranpō* physicians had become the public policy of the Japanese state.

ONE

Confronting Smallpox

At the beginning of the nineteenth century, smallpox was a force to be reckoned with—a universal disease and the world's most reliable killer. The virus that causes smallpox, *Variola major*, was a tireless migrant that moved continuously from place to place in search of susceptible human hosts to infect. Because a human host provided only a temporary residence for *V. major*, the death or recovery of its host meant that the virus had to move on in search of a new one. Hence, the smallpox virus thrived in cities and other places where the number of human hosts was large or where a high birth rate produced new hosts to accommodate the peripatetic virus. In such places, smallpox became an endemic disease that circulated continuously from one susceptible human host to another. World population growth and increases in the number and size of cities eventually created environments in which the smallpox virus could sustain itself indefinitely.[1]

In ancient times, the migrations of the variola virus were contained within separate spheres of contact that connected the great civilizations of the Old World. Human migrations of all sorts—interregional trade, wars, and expansion across frontiers—facilitated the spread of the smallpox virus to populations where smallpox was unknown and where every living person was a susceptible host. A dramatic transmission of the variola virus occurred with the discovery of the Western Hemisphere by Europeans. The human migrations that followed allowed *V. major* to make a transoceanic leap to the New World, where it found large new populations to infect, and these areas experienced massive depopulation from smallpox. In societies that experienced regular exposure to smallpox, the case-fatality rate was about 25 percent; however, in societies that encountered smallpox infrequently, the rate was much higher. When a high proportion of the population was stricken within a short period of time, few healthy individuals remained to care for large numbers of desperately ill people, and the death rate rose as a result.

In early modern times, as long-distance trade expanded to connect virtually all regions of the world, the smallpox virus was able to establish a global migratory sphere. *V. major* traveled by land and by sea, a frequent companion of its human host. By the eighteenth century, smallpox had become a universal disease that afflicted societies everywhere. Survivors of smallpox acquired lifetime immunity to the disease; hence, in densely settled populations where smallpox was endemic, it soon became a disease of children. Virtually all living adults were smallpox survivors, many of whom bore the hideous, disfiguring scars that were the telltale mark of the disease. High smallpox mortality rates could check population growth in places where the disease was endemic, but because most adults were immune, smallpox only rarely challenged political and social stability in those places.

By contrast, communities with small, scattered populations that had few contacts with the world's population centers could avoid exposure to smallpox for long periods. However, when the variola virus did strike and a large proportion of the population was infected, the political, social, and demographic effects could be devastating. In addition to virgin populations experiencing smallpox for the first time, nomadic communities and pastoral peoples who moved from place to place on the fringes of settled, agrarian societies were especially vulnerable. They too suffered unusually high mortality rates from smallpox when they came in contact with their more settled neighbors.

As the migratory sphere of *V. major* expanded and the incidence of smallpox cases increased, smallpox apparently became a more virulent disease. Certainly, seventeenth-century European observers believed that smallpox was a more serious disease than it had been in earlier times. Given the absence of case-fatality statistics, it is not possible to confirm this observation, but the annual bills of mortality for London, which began to be published in 1629, indicate that smallpox was already a major cause of death and increasingly caused a larger proportion of all deaths.[2] This trend was observed in the eighteenth century as well. Genevieve Miller has referred to smallpox as "a formidable new scourge" that was "taking the place of old enemies like the plague. . . ."[3] It was common wisdom not to count one's children until they had survived smallpox.

What could be done? Apart from invoking divine protection, the time-honored methods of combatting smallpox were flight and isolation. But however effective these methods might be in the short run, where smallpox was endemic, they only postponed the inevitable. With the knowledge that exposure to smallpox was virtually certain, that no effective treatment existed, and that death or disfigurement were likely outcomes, two options presented themselves: to wait for smallpox to strike and hope for the best, or to deliberately expose one's children to smallpox under the most favorable circumstances possible. Interest in the latter option led to experimentation with a variety of techniques known as variolation. Before either the term or the concept of immunization had been formulated, variolation techniques were granting lifelong immunity to smallpox.

VARIOLATION

The purpose of variolation was to bring children safely through the ordeal of smallpox. The most primitive practice was simply to expose an uninfected person to a person with a mild case of smallpox; or, alternatively, to wrap a person in blankets or garments that recently had been worn by someone with a mild case. Casual exposure to smallpox could be accomplished without medical assistance, and in many parts of the world where smallpox was endemic, deliberate exposure was a rite of passage orchestrated by parents whose children had not yet had the disease.[4] This practice was not without risk. Exposure to someone with even a relatively mild case was a dangerous gamble; a benign outcome was by no means insured. Taking such a risk would have been unthinkable had not the likelihood of contracting an even more virulent case of smallpox by natural means been so great.

What initially had been a simple folk remedy eventually developed into a highly sophisticated medical technique. Because of the danger involved, variolation was used most often when smallpox was epidemic and known to be circulating nearby. The imminent threat of exposure forced an immediate choice between naturally acquired smallpox and carefully induced smallpox. While deliberate exposure to mild cases of smallpox was being practiced in many communities throughout the world, more sophisticated variolation techniques were being developed in China and Turkey—two large population centers where smallpox was an endemic disease. Knowledge of these Chinese and Turkish techniques spread slowly, first by word of mouth or demonstration and later through texts disseminated and translated into different languages.[5]

Chinese-Style Variolation

Evidence of the practice of variolation can be clearly identified in China by the sixteenth century. Initially a technique used by lay or folk practitioners, variolation subsequently was adopted by adherents of the Chinese Fever School of South China. Despite the fact that medical ideas associated with the Fever School were frowned upon by proponents of the more orthodox medical theories of North China, physicians in the South promoted variolation with considerable success. Variolation became a medical specialty, and physicians developed specific techniques, which they guarded jealously. Some physicians used smallpox lymph, the liquid substance contained in the smallpox vesicle, as the infecting agent; others used dried smallpox scabs that had been ground into a powder. In both cases, they recognized that it was essential to preserve the vitality of the variola virus, because if the virus died, immunization against smallpox would fail.

Chinese variolation simulated the way smallpox was acquired naturally, by breathing airborne droplets of the virus through the nasal passages and into the lungs. The variolator would collect the virus from a person infected with smallpox when the infective capacity of the virus was considered ideal, around the eighth day in the course of the disease. The virus would then be weakened, or attenuated, by storing it in a cool, dark place for several days or even several months. The Chinese learned that smallpox lymph lost its vitality quickly in hot weather, whereas when the virus was collected and stored as scabs, the virus remained viable for much longer periods. In the seventeenth and eighteenth centuries the "dry" or "nasal insufflation" method of variolation came to be widely used in China. Smallpox scabs were ground into a powder and blown through a tube inserted into a child's nostril—the right nostril if the child was a boy and the left nostril if a girl.

A compelling advantage of variolation over naturally acquired smallpox was that the variola virus could be administered to a healthy person who then would be isolated from other individuals. This assured that the person variolated would not inadvertently spread smallpox to others. Eighteenth-century Chinese physicians produced highly sophisticated variolation techniques; an extensive medical literature recommending specific ways to collect, attenuate, and store the variola virus; and instructions on how to perform the procedure.[6] Eventually a consensus developed that fewer children died from variolation than from naturally acquired smallpox.

In the second half of the seventeenth century, under the patronage of China's Manchu rulers, Chinese-style variolation spread to North China. The Manchu people, like other inhabitants of the Northeast Asian steppe, encountered smallpox only rarely in their homeland, which meant that adults were as susceptible as children to the disease. When the Manchus invaded China in 1644, they already knew about the threat of smallpox, because pre-conquest Manchu missions to China had witnessed the loss to smallpox of many of their members. The Manchu rulers of the Qing Dynasty (1644-1911) devised a biopolitical strategy during their conquest of China, and afterward, to counteract this vulnerability by choosing their leaders and troops from among Manchu tribesmen who had already had smallpox. Despite this cautious approach, the first Qing Emperor, Shunzhi (1638-1661, r. 1644-1661) died of smallpox at age twenty-three. His successor, the Kangxi Emperor (1654-1722, r. 1662-1722), was chosen over an older brother, because Kangxi had survived smallpox and was known to be immune.[7] Manchu vulnerability, especially in the early part of the dynasty, meant that under the Qing, smallpox prevention became state policy, and variolation was officially recognized as the most effective way to immunize Manchu government officials and members of the military.[8]

How far the practice of variolation spread beyond the Qing territories is less clear. Published literature on variolation was available to those who could read Chinese, which would have included Korean physicians whose medical tradition was derived from the Chinese. Korean diplomatic missions came regularly to China, and if variolation were an accepted medical tradition at the Qing court, it seems likely that Korean physicians would have learned about it and used it as well.

Japan, on the other hand, avoided contact with China in the seventeenth century, but during the last half-century of Ming rule (1368–1644), many Chinese physicians fled from South China to Japan to escape political turmoil. They brought their knowledge of Chinese-style variolation with them; and they became permanent residents, settled into the Chinese merchant community in Nagasaki, and often took Japanese names. Prominent among these medical immigrants were physicians affiliated with the Chinese Fever School who had practiced variolation before coming to Japan.[9] Early seventeenth-century Japanese sources are silent on the subject of variolation; however, it seems unlikely that the Chinese physicians who took up residence in Nagasaki would have abandoned such a useful practice.

Initially, at least, Chinese immigrant-physicians formed an influential medical community in Nagasaki, and the ideas of the Chinese Fever School formed the basis for the Japanese Kōseiha School, which dominated Japanese medical thinking during the early Edo period. Dai Manquang, an expert Chinese variolator, had published ten volumes devoted to the pathology and variolation of smallpox before he emigrated from China to Japan in 1653. The Tokugawa government sent physicians from Edo to Nagasaki to study under Dai, and to create a new medical specialty devoted to the study and treatment of smallpox.[10] This interest in variolation on the part of the Edo government seems to have lapsed, because there is little evidence of the dissemination of knowledge about Chinese-style variolation to other parts of Japan. To deliberately infect a child with smallpox required a firm belief that induced smallpox was a better option than naturally acquired smallpox. Possibly no prominent school of medical thought in Japan became a strong advocate of this view. The folk custom of deliberately exposing children to mild cases of smallpox was used in Japan,[11] but, as will be discussed below, not until the late eighteenth century did information about Chinese-style variolation begin to attract the attention of practicing Japanese physicians.

Marta E. Hanson has observed that Chinese medical knowledge was transmitted westward to Russia and other European countries during the seventeenth century by means of Jesuit translations of Chinese medical texts.[12] It is not clear how far this information spread; however, in the early eighteenth century, the Royal Society of London received information about Chinese-style variolation from an English employee of the East India Company who had witnessed the procedure in China. In a letter dated January 5, 1700, Joseph Lister described the Chinese insufflation method as a technique that involved "opening the pustules of one who has the Small Pox ripe upon them and drying up the Matter with a little Cotton, which they preserve in a close box, & afterwards put it up the nostrils of those they would infect."[13] He thought that this technique might only be practicable "in these parts," but the advantage, he pointed out, was that a child could be prepared for the illness at the most appropriate age and season.[14] Even so, despite the earlier arrival of information about Chinese-style variolation, it was the Turkish method that gained prominence in Britain and Western Europe.[15]

Turkish-Style Variolation

The variolation technique that developed around the eastern Mediterranean, in the cosmopolitan centers of Greece and Turkey, had the same purpose as Chinese variolation: to induce a mild case of smallpox and insure future immunity. Unlike the Chinese inhalation method, which introduced the infection to internal organs through the respiratory system, Turkish-style variolation was a surgical technique introduced through the skin of the recipient. The variolator inserted live variola virus—ideally fresh lymph taken directly from a smallpox vesicle—into one or more scratches or incisions made in the skin. The Turkish variolation technique was called inoculation.

The Royal Society of London was an important forum for considering new medical and scientific knowledge. Its members collected information and presented papers on a wide range of subjects that physicians and scientists from around the world sent to members of the Society.[16] Early in the eighteenth century, the Royal Society received reports from two Italian physicians about a practice of "transplanting" smallpox that was used in Constantinople. Constantinople was an international entrepôt where Greek, Italian, Dutch, French, and English diplomats and businessmen resided for extended periods of time. Two Italian physicians, Emanuele Timoni and Jacob Pylarini, both of whom had medical degrees from the University of Padua, had personally observed inoculation in Constantinople. The papers they submitted to the Royal Society described what they referred to as "Turkish inoculation." Timoni's paper was published in the Society's journal, *Philosophical Transactions,* in 1714; Pylarini's paper, which already had been published in Venice in late 1715, was reprinted in the *Philosophical Transactions* the following spring.[17]

Meanwhile, Britons who were living in Constantinople were having their own children inoculated (variolated). The secretary to the British ambassador had his two sons inoculated before returning to London in 1716. And in March 1717, Lady Mary Wortley Montagu, the wife of the subsequent British ambassador, convinced Charles Maitland, the Scottish surgeon who was serving at the British embassy in Constantinople, to inoculate her young son, Edward Montague.[18] She clearly was pleased with the result, because she wrote to a friend in England to say that when she returned to London she intended to introduce the "useful invention" of "ingrafting of the smallpox into fashion in England."[19]

Lady Mary got her chance to do just that when she returned to London in 1721. An unusually severe smallpox epidemic struck the city that year, and she asked Charles Maitland to inoculate her young daughter. Maitland complied with great reluctance, and only after Lady Mary agreed to have other physicians present to serve as witnesses. The practice of requiring witnesses to be present when new, potentially life-threatening medical technologies were being tried and the outcome was uncertain was not uncommon. Witnesses could attest to the professionalism of the physician and the willingness of the parents to have their child undergo the procedure; they could also help disseminate news of good or bad outcomes by recounting later what they had observed.

The inoculation of Lady Montagu's daughter took place in April 1721, with three witnesses from the Royal College of Physicians in attendance. One witness, Dr. James Keith, was so impressed by the mildness of the disease that followed that he had Maitland inoculate his only surviving child, a six-year-old son. James Keith's other children had all died of smallpox.[20] At the time, there was no public report of this privately commissioned inoculation and its success, but word circulated in aristocratic and professional circles.

Four months later, a royal commission ordered Charles Maitland to conduct a medical trial by inoculating six condemned prisoners. Sir Hans Sloane and Dr. John George Steigherthal, as royal physicians representing the king, supervised the inoculations at Newgate prison. Approximately twenty-five physicians, surgeons, and apothecaries, and prominent members of the Royal College of Physicians and the Royal Society, were additional witnesses at the trial. Other interested physicians were allowed to visit the prison daily to monitor the progress of the prisoners—all of whom recovered, were pardoned, and then released. These proceedings were made public and reported in the London newspapers.[21]

It was an auspicious beginning for Turkish-style variolation in England. A year after the public trial on condemned prisoners, Charles Maitland would inoculate the younger children of the royal family, and it was not long before English physicians and lay practitioners were "inoculating the smallpox" in communities throughout the British Isles.[22] Inoculation trials would continue to test the effectiveness and safety of variolation, but the early involvement of King and Council, the Royal Society, and the Royal College of Physicians—the primary institutions of Britain's scientific community—set a standard for consultation between the political and scientific leadership in Britain.

It is interesting to note that some of the earliest promoters of inoculation were lay people. Not all reports about the benefits of variolation came from physicians, or from China and Constantinople. Cotton Mather, a well-known preacher who lived in Boston, had learned about African variolation from his household slave, Onisemus, a native of Tripoli.[23] As early as 1716, Mather wrote to Dr. John Woodward, a Fellow of the Royal Society, to inquire why the practice had not been tried in England. He explained that he would try variolation himself the next time smallpox was prevalent in Boston, but he must wait because at present there was no smallpox virus available to perform the procedure. The population of Boston at that time was too small to support endemic smallpox. Significantly, neither Lady Mary nor Cotton Mather, who independently sponsored the introduction of variolation in Britain and the American colonies, respectively, was a physician.

In England, where smallpox virus was almost always available, English physicians initially were reluctant to perform variolation. But forces were at work to change this. Miller has argued that eighteenth-century Enlightenment ideas made Europeans more open to foreign solutions to common problems. No one doubted that smallpox was a common and serious problem, and the increasing virulence of this disease gained the attention of individual physicians and medical societies. In 1727, Dr. John Arbuthnot in his Harveian Oration to the Royal College of Physicians called the need for physicians to make smallpox less hazardous one of the most urgent medical problems of the day. He suggested to his fellow physicians that Turkish-style variolation was "an Eastern innovation" well worth investigating.[24]

Meanwhile, inoculation trials were being conducted privately and publicly in various parts of Europe, and physicians were beginning to disseminate their diverse opinions about "inoculating the smallpox" across national borders. European universities and scientific societies allowed physicians, scientists, and governments to collect and share ideas as they sought effective ways to deal with the accelerating problem of smallpox mortality, and these institutions greatly facilitated the transmission of medical knowledge between Western countries. Despite the fact that these were national institutions, they were international in terms of their interests and membership. Not only were they major repositories of scientific information contributed from all over the world, but individuals were admitted to membership on the basis of their contribution to the advancement of scientific knowledge, not on the basis of national origin. The eighteenth century was an age of scientific exploration: scientists, medical men, traders, explorers, and travelers reported their findings in all sorts of ways—casually by word of mouth, and more formally through lectures, letters, books, and articles published in newspapers and popular and scientific journals.

The translation and publication of important medical texts into the vernacular European languages was a boon to the transmission of new medical knowledge. Medicine was an international field in which physicians frequently trained with professors in universities and hospitals in countries other than their own. The career of Lorenz Heister (1683–1758), an eminent German physician and surgeon, exemplifies the extent to which broad international medical training contributed to the dissemination of medical advances in the eighteenth century.

In the preface to his influential book *Chirurgie*,[25] Heister reviewed the course of his own training as follows:

> After having studied *Physic* . . . above four years in our German Universities, my Affections, being strongest for *Anatomy* and *Surgery*, led me to the then celebrated Professors Ruysch and Raw at *Amsterdam* in the Year 1706. . . . [T]here being at that time a sharp war in *Flanders* betwixt the *French* and *Dutch*, . . . in the Year 1707, I went from *Holland* to the *Dutch* Camp in *Brabant*, that I might inspect and observe the Practice of the *English*, *Dutch*, and *German* Surgeons, who there attended. [I]n autumn I went from *Brabant* to *Leyden*, and spent the whole Winter in attending the Lectures of the then celebrated Professors in that University, Bidloo, Albinus senior, and Boerhaave; and thus I continued till the Beginning of the Summer 1708.[26]

Following this period as an itinerant student in the medical centers of Europe, Heister became a military surgeon in the Dutch army and developed revolutionary new techniques for dealing with battlefield wounds. Appointed Professor of Anatomy and Surgery at the University of Altdorf in the Republic of Nurnberg, he soon obtained leave to tour universities and hospitals in Great Britain where he collected "every thing new in the several Branches of Physic."[27] Heister then returned to his professorship in Nurnberg, where he gave lectures and published books in Latin. But he chose quite purposefully to publish *Chirurgie* in German: "considering the Ignorance of our German Surgeons, . . . it being chiefly composed and intended for them, I now judged it would be more useful to print . . . in our native German. . . ."[28]

The first edition of *Chirurgie* was published in German in Nurnberg in 1719. Successive German editions were published in 1724, 1743, 1752, and 1753; a Latin edition was published in Amsterdam in 1738, a Dutch edition in 1741, and eight English editions were published between 1740 and 1759.

During Lorenz Heister's lifetime, variolation was just beginning to gain adherents, but Heister advocated inoculation with the variola virus long before the technique was generally accepted by European physicians more generally. He based his assessment of the efficacy of inoculation largely on the reports of English physicians. In Chapter XV of *Chirurgie*, Heister gave explicit instructions on how to perform inoculation. This early contribution, reproduced below, to debates over the benefits of variolation leaves no doubt that Heister favored the technique of "inoculating the smallpox."

Of INOCULATION *for the* SMALL POX

I. The Art of engrafting or propagating the Small Pox by Incision or Inoculation has been an Operation equally famous in all Nations . . . ; and therefore we shall, for the sake of Beginners, describe the Process of it, which under proper Circumstances may be of great Service to Mankind.

II. The Design of this Operation is to communicate by Art a milder Species of the Small Pox to the Infant or adult Patient, than that received by the natural Infection, and this by engrafting some of the variolous Matter; in order to which a small Incision is to be first made with a Scalpel or Lancet through the Skin of the Arm, and having inserted a small Particle of the purulent Matter taken from a mild kind of the Pock, the little Wound is then to be dressed with some dry Lint, and covered with a Plaster. After the Operation the Patient must constantly keep to his Chamber, the Air of which should be moderately warm, and his Diet regulated by some prudent Physician, by which means the Disorder will shew itself in about seven or eight Days, without any malignant Symptoms; . . . it usually runs gently through its several Stages. When the Patient has once had the Disorder this way, though ever so mild, we are assured by Experience that they never have it again; and therefore the Opinion of those seems to be well grounded who think the Propagation of the Small Pox by Inoculation might be of general Use and Benefit to Mankind, in preserving the Lives of some, and the most important Members of others, as the Face, Eyes, Hearing, Viscera, &c.[29]

The fact that an internationally respected physician and surgeon could communicate support for a new medical technology through professional channels did not mean that inoculation became a general practice. While variolation drew strong support from some professional, intellectual, and aristocratic groups, strong opposition continued from a large segment of the medical profession, from religious groups, and from the lower classes. Even among those who accepted that the risk of dying from variolation might be lower than that of dying from natural smallpox, few wished to face that risk until smallpox was epidemic and its threat was imminent.

VARIOLATION IN JAPAN

Japan had suffered from smallpox since ancient times. One of the world's earliest accounts of a smallpox epidemic can be found in an entry in the *Nihongi* (*Chronicles of Japan*) for the year AD 585.[30] Detailed accounts of a severe smallpox epidemic in 735–737 state that the disease afflicted people of all ages,[31] indicating that few people living at the time had been exposed to smallpox previously. By the twelfth century, however, contemporary accounts state that smallpox was infecting primarily the youngest members of the population, suggesting that smallpox was becoming an endemic disease in Japan. By the fifteenth century, smallpox had clearly become a disease of Japanese children.[32] Seventeenth-century Dutch reports confirm the prevalence of smallpox in the port city of Nagasaki: ". . . many people are dying in Nagasaki, sometimes 30, 40, 50, yea even 67 people are being buried on a day, mainly young children dying from smallpox."[33] By the eighteenth century, as in Europe, smallpox had become a devastating disease of children. In even the remote regions of Hida Province, in the mountains of central Japan, smallpox was epidemic every three to four years, and claimed the lives of 20 percent of all children born, most of them before the age of five.[34]

Despite the severity of smallpox in eighteenth-century Japan and the proximity of China, where variolation had been practiced for at least two centuries, and despite the fact that Japanese physicians had learned of variolation from Chinese physicians in Nagasaki more than a century earlier, variolation was not generally accepted practice in Japan. However, during the eighteenth century, two separate attempts to introduce Chinese-style and Turkish-style variolation indicate increasing interest in the procedure.

In 1744, a Chinese merchant named Li Jen-shan, a dealer in Chinese and European goods, who happened to be in Nagasaki during a smallpox epidemic, told the Nagasaki Governor (*machi bugyō*), Matsunami Heizaemon, about the Chinese method of variolation. Li was asked to explain the method to two Ōmura domain physicians, who then were ordered to perform the procedure on twenty Nagasaki prostitutes.[35] Li's instructions were recorded in a Japanese treatise entitled *Li Jen-shan no shutō sho* (*Li Jen-shan's Treatise on Variolation*).[36]

Li's personal communication about Chinese variolation was followed by additional information coming from China. A comprehensive medical encyclopedia entitled *Yi zong jin jian* (*The Official Compilation: The Golden Mirror of Medicine*) arrived in Japan in 1752. First published in Peking a decade earlier, this text, consisting of ninety chapters, was a compilation of many earlier texts. *Yi zong jin jian* represented a synthesis of Chinese medicine at the time.[37] The text contains two early treatises on smallpox believed to have been in circulation well before 1740. Chang Chia-feng believes these texts may be the earliest surviving Chinese variolation treatises of the Qing period.[38] The Japanese reading of the Chinese title is *Isō kinkan*. In 1778, the section on Chinese-style variolation was excerpted and published separately as *Shutō shinpō* (*A New Way to Implant Smallpox*).

It had taken thirty years for a Chinese text that contained important information about smallpox prevention to attract much attention in Japan. *Shutō shinpō* became the standard manual in Japan on how to use Chinese-style variolation to immunize children against smallpox.[39] Importing Chinese medical books was common practice, but it is not clear how the texts to be imported were chosen. Li Jen-shan's personal communication of information about Chinese-style variolation seems to have created little interest, but it may be that his reports about Chinese-style variolation prompted requests for other Chinese medical writings on the subject, which came later.

Only one of the four methods described in *Isō kinkan*—the Chinese nasal insufflation, or dry, method—was used to any extent in Japan.[40] The instructions were to dry and store smallpox crusts under specified conditions designed to weaken the virus; the smallpox crusts were pulverized into a powder, which then was blown through a tube into a child's nostril. The Japanese called this technique *jintō sesshu or jintō shutō*; both terms mean "implanting human smallpox." The infective agent—*Variola major*, in the form of lymph or attenuated scabs—was called *byō* or "seed."[41]

In the final decade of the eighteenth century, A. L. Bernardus Keller, resident physician at the Dutch Factory from 1790–1795, introduced the surgical, Turkish-style variolation at Dejima.[42] Using a lancet to insert live smallpox lymph into small wounds in the arms of several Japanese children, he was able to execute four successful inoculations. Keller, like others who practiced Turkish-style variolation, recommended that smallpox lymph be used for inoculation and that it be taken directly from a person with a mild case of smallpox. In 1794, when Keller went on the court journey to Edo with the Dutch Factory personnel to pay tribute to the shogun, he met with physicians interested in Western-style (*ranpō*) medicine.[43] Among those he met in Edo were two *rangaku* scholars, Katsuragawa Hōshu, physician to the shogun, and Ōtsuki Gentaku, the physician who is regarded as the founder of the *rangaku*, or Dutch learning, movement. Both of these men would write treatises about Western-style variolation.[44]

Variolation would eventually attract the attention of a few Japanese physicians, some of whom experimented with various ways of attenuating the virus and infecting recipients. However, neither Chinese-style nor Turkish-style variolation seemed to catch on in Japan as it had in China and parts of the West. Variolation failed to gain official support, and there is little evidence to suggest that it was widely used by private medical practitioners. If we ask why Japan's medical community and government officials failed to adopt an effective technique that was being used successfully to contain smallpox in China, the answer must be speculative, but it was not because the smallpox virus was not always present. The Nagasaki Governor who ordered variolation trials had clearly thought that the information brought by the Chinese merchant, Li Jen-shan, was of sufficient importance to record and to test on humans. But how to proceed further?

There seem to have been few channels through which individuals, even high-ranking officials like the Nagasaki *machi bugyō*, who had been appointed by the Tokugawa shogun, could disseminate useful medical information throughout Japan. The problem was not the Chinese source of the information: Chinese medicine was the orthodox medical tradition in Japan, and Japanese physicians were accustomed to reading Chinese medical texts and adopting Chinese medical practices. The practice of their profession depended upon their being able to do so. But in the Tokugawa period, information from all foreign sources—Chinese and Western—was transmitted to Japan through Nagasaki. Nagasaki was not considered as a place of learning, nor was it yet the specialized center for the study of Western medicine that it would become in the nineteenth century. But the fact that Nagasaki was the source of foreign knowledge, and the place where those who were most proficient in Dutch lived, meant that the city became a magnet for individuals interested in studying about the West.

A high proportion of individuals who went to Nagasaki to study were physicians. Although incentives for transmitting information about practical medical techniques like Chinese-style and Turkish-style variolation did not exist in eighteenth-century Japan, by the end of the century, private, personal, and informal networks emanating from Nagasaki were beginning to develop. Because medicine was a hereditary occupation, medical knowledge was passed down from one generation to the next through established medical lineages, and innovative medical therapies were usually kept secret. However, newcomers to medical practice had no family secrets to protect. Medicine offered one of the best avenues of upward mobility in Tokugawa Japan, and during the late eighteenth and early nineteenth centuries, many young men entered medicine from commoner and lower samurai ranks.

One of these newcomers was Ogata Shunsaku (1748–1810), the second son in a samurai family in Kyushu, who was adopted by a local physician named Ogata Gensai. Gensai sent Shunsaku to Nagasaki to study with Yoshio Kōzaemon (1842–1800), a physician who practiced and taught therapies and techniques based on Western- or Dutch-style (*ranpō*) medicine. The Yoshio family was one of the official interpreter lineages that had served the Edo *bakufu* as Nagasaki interpreters since the mid-seventeenth century. Trained to read Dutch for the purpose of translating Dutch commercial documents, more than a few members of the Yoshio family also learned about Western-style surgery from the European physicians attached to the Dutch Factory. Interested physicians and students engaged these Japanese interpreter-physicians to teach them the Dutch language and Western medical techniques for a fee.

While studying with Yoshio Kōzaemon in Nagasaki, Ogata Shunsaku discovered and made a copy of the Chinese-style variolation treatise called *Shutō shinpō*. Upon leaving Nagasaki, Shunsaku opened a medical practice in

Akitsuki domain, Chikuzen Province, and in 1789 he was appointed to an official post as domain physician. When a severe smallpox epidemic broke out that year, he decided to try the Chinese nasal insufflation method that he had read about in *Shutō shinpō*. First, he variolated the daughter of a local merchant and then the children of other domain physicians. Then, having encountered no problems, Shunsaku began to variolate children elsewhere in the domain without, he claimed, a single death. In 1790, convinced that Chinese-style variolation should be used to prevent the more serious infections caused by natural smallpox, Shunsaku traveled to Kyoto, Osaka, and Edo to report his successes and to promote the practice of Chinese-style variolation in those cities.[45]

After his return to Akitsuki, Ogata Shunsaku opened a school to teach his method to others, and in 1793 he wrote a treatise documenting his experiences using the Chinese variolation technique. The treatise, *Shutō hitsu jun ben* (*The Need for Variolation*), suggests several ways to improve and standardize the Chinese procedure. The age and condition of the *byō* (the variola virus), Shunsaku explained, was a matter of the greatest importance. Smallpox crusts should be collected from an infected person on the eleventh day of illness and stored in a sealed ceramic container in a cool, dark place. How long the crusts could be stored and remain effective depended upon the season of the year; he warned their effectiveness would last for fifty days in winter but only thirty days in summer. This observation is consistent with what later became known about the sensitivity of the smallpox virus to heat.[46]

Although Ogata Shunsaku was acquainted with the Dutch physician Bernardus Keller, there is no evidence that he ever tried to use or promote Western-style variolation. That may have been because Chinese-style variolation had distinct advantages in places like Kyushu with its hot, moist climate. Smallpox lymph did not remain viable very long, whereas, as Shunsaku claimed, smallpox crusts could be stored for fairly long periods. Moreover, as noted above, even if crusts were no more effective than lymph, the fact that they could be stored and reconstituted allowed physicians to decide the most propitious time to variolate a patient. And it was not necessary always to have an infected smallpox donor on hand to provide live smallpox virus on a specific day of the infection.

Shunsaku was among the first of many Japanese physicians to discover that foreign physicians were experimenting with variolation techniques to prevent smallpox and to take matters into his own hands. He was certainly among the first to write about it. His personal efforts to promote Chinese-style variolation seem to have had little impact beyond his own domain, but there is no way to assess whether his writings or the physicians with whom he shared his experiences took up the practice of variolation.

Without medical societies and journals to report, discuss, and test the efficacy of variolation, individual physicians continued to seek ideas and instruction from foreign medical books. Like Ogata Shunsaku, they used what they had learned to experiment on their own patients. It would be another half-century before the physicians who became staunch advocates of medical techniques to contain smallpox were in a position to collaborate on a nation-wide scale.

*   *   *

In the 1790s, as Ogata Shunsaku was experimenting with Chinese-style variolation in Japan, an English physician who practiced medicine in the dairy farming region of Gloucestershire was experimenting with a technique that would replace variolation. Having observed that dairy workers who had been infected with the disease of cowpox were spared subsequent infection with smallpox, Edward Jenner set out to prove a cause-and-effect relationship between the two observations. The results of Jenner's experiments were published before the end of the century and would initiate a revolution in medicine.

Jenner's Cowpox Vaccine

In 1798, on the eve of the publication of his first treatise on the cowpox, Edward Jenner wrote to C. H. Parry, M.D., a friend and colleague living in Bath:

> My Dear Friend,
>   In the present age of scientific investigation, it is remarkable that a disease of so peculiar a nature as the Cow Pox, which has appeared in this and some of the neighbouring counties for such a series of years, should so long have escaped particular attention. Finding the prevailing notions on the subject, both among men of our profession and others, extremely vague and indeterminate, and conceiving that facts might appear at once curious and useful, I have instituted as strict an inquiry into the causes and effects of this singular malady as local circumstances would admit.
>   The following pages are the result, which, from motives of the most affectionate regard, are dedicated to you, by
>
>
>
> Your sincere Friend,
> EDWARD JENNER
> Berkeley, Gloucestershire
> June 21st, 1798[1]
>
>

The "following pages" to which Jenner referred were a draft of his treatise, *An Inquiry into the Causes and Effects of the Variolae Vaccinae, a Disease Discovered in some of the Western Counties of England, Particularly Gloucestershire, and Known by the Name of the Cow Pox* (henceforth *Inquiry*). But *Inquiry* was no ordinary treatise about a peculiar disease of cattle, and Jenner knew it. Neither Jenner's letter nor the modest, if lengthy, title of his treatise provides the slightest hint of the revolutionary and global impact his *Inquiry* would have on medicine, science, and society. Nor does it convey any sense of the controversies his claim would provoke up to the present day.

Born in Berkeley, Gloucestershire, England, in 1743, Edward Jenner was the son of a clergyman and the youngest child in a large family. His parents died when he was young, and he was raised by his older siblings. Starting in childhood, Jenner was interested in natural history and intrigued by the life cycles of animals and birds in the neighboring countryside. Jenner's childhood interests continued after he took up the study of medicine, and they developed further under the tutelage of his mentor, the famous London anatomist, surgeon, and scientist, John Hunter. Hunter encouraged Jenner "to seek the underlying causes of disease in both animals and humans by dissection and by comparing individual case histories."[2] After Jenner returned to Gloucestershire to practice medicine, he continued to collaborate with Hunter on a wide range of scientific and medical experiments that involved animals, such as the hedgehog, which had to be conducted in the countryside. Jenner investigated the physiology of hibernating animals and the flight patterns of migrating birds, and in 1789 he astonished the scientific community with a highly original paper on the predatory nesting habits of the cuckoo.[3] This paper, which led to his election as a Fellow of the Royal Society on February 25, 1789, was translated and published in Italian and French in 1791.[4]

THE COWPOX VIRUS

In eighteenth-century England, cowpox was a fairly common disease that afflicted cattle in some but not all years. In the dairy farming country of Gloucestershire, milkmaids or anyone who handled infected cows might also become infected, especially if they had cuts or scratches on their hands. They broke out in pocks, or lesions, that resembled the pocks on the udders of the cows. Cowpox was not a serious disease when acquired by humans in this way. Besides the pocks that began to emerge within a few days of exposure, the usual symptoms were a slight fever and malaise lasting a day or two. The pocks, when they appeared, filled with a liquid that thickened and then dried up within a week to ten days. Compared to the more virulent small-pox, the course of the disease of cowpox was exceedingly mild in humans.

Jenner was in his fifties when he began seriously to investigate possible relationships between the disease of cattle known as "cow pox," the equine disease called "horse pox," and the human disease of "small pox." Given his knowledge of the culture of dairy farming and his interest in natural history, Jenner's fascination with the "peculiar" disease of cowpox would have sur-prised few who knew him. They might, however, have been surprised by the energy and tenacity with which he turned this fascination into a lifelong crusade to eradicate the devastating disease of smallpox.

Jenner's *Inquiry* made the boldest of claims: once a person was infected with cowpox, he or she would no longer be susceptible to smallpox. To ini-tiate his discussion of the relationship between cowpox and smallpox, Jenner elevated the status of cowpox by giving the disease a proper binomial Latin-Linnaean name: *Variolae vaccinae*. He could then discuss it on the same plane as *Variola major*, the medical-scientific name for smallpox. The term *vaccinae* was derived from the Latin word *vacca*, for cow. Jenner was not the first to ob-serve that individuals who once had been infected with cowpox seemed to be resistant, or immune, to smallpox.[5] He was, however, the first to devise and carry out a series of experiments designed to prove it; the first to submit the evidence to the scientific community for peer review; and the first to attempt to convince others, by every means at his disposal, that his claim was valid.

In the short introduction to his *Inquiry*, Jenner is supremely confident:

> What renders the Cow-pox virus so extremely singular, is, that the person who has been thus affected [infected] is forever secure from the infection of the Small Pox; neither exposure to the variolous effluvia, nor the insertion of the matter into the skin, producing this distemper [smallpox].
>
> In support of so extraordinary a fact, I shall lay before my Reader a great number of instances.[6]

And he proceeded to do just that. Following a brief introduction, Jenner pre-sented twenty-three case histories. He began with first-hand accounts from individuals who had been infected with cowpox at some time in the past, and despite repeated exposure to smallpox, failed to contract the latter disease.

Jenner's first case was John Merret, a farmer who had been infected with cowpox in 1770 while working for the Earl of Berkeley. In April 1797, in anticipation of an approaching smallpox epidemic, there was a general inoculation (variolation) of the population of Berkeley. Merret was variolated with the rest of his family, but the variolation did not "take"; he failed to experience any of the usual symptoms following smallpox inoculation. Jenner also variolated Merret, but failed to produce the symptoms characteristic of smallpox: "[T]hough the variolous matter was repeatedly inserted into his arm, I found it impracticable to infect him with it. . . . During the whole time that his family had the Small Pox, one of whom had it very full, he remained in the house with them, but received no injury from exposure to the contagion."[7]

In a succession of similar case histories, Jenner explains the circumstances in which various local individuals had become infected with cowpox. He then tells how he variolated each person with smallpox matter to see if he or she would contract smallpox. To this point, Jenner's case studies simply documented the subsequent histories of people who accidentally had caught cowpox from infected cows. When he inoculated these same individuals with smallpox lymph many years later, and when they failed to show any signs of smallpox, Jenner concluded that the earlier cowpox infection was still protecting them from smallpox.

Had Jenner stopped his experiments at this juncture, he would have done little more than document what others before him had observed. With Cases 16 and 17, however, Jenner ventured onto new terrain:

> Sarah Nelmes, a dairy maid at a Farmer's near this place, was infected with the Cow Pox from her Master's cows in May, 1796. She received the infection on a part of the hand which had been previously in a slight degree injured by a scratch from a thorn. A large pustulous sore and the usual symptoms accompanying the disease were produced in consequence. The pustule was so expressive of the true character of the Cow Pox, as it commonly appears upon the hand, that I have given a representation of it in the annexed plate.[8]

The *Inquiry* displays a full-page colored plate to illustrate "the true character" of the cowpox pustule on Sarah Nelmes's arm. This illustration represented the precise appearance of the cowpox pustule to depict "a condition never seen before."[9] As Jenner explained, the illustration was not a true representation but a composite intended to show two different stages of the disease. "The pustule on the finger shews the disease in an earlier stage. It did not actually appear on the hand of this young woman, but was taken from that of another, and is annexed for the purpose of representing the malady after it has newly appeared."[10]

The next step in Jenner's investigation was to inoculate a young local boy, James Phipps, who had not yet had smallpox, with lymph taken from the pock on the arm of Sarah Nelmes:

> The more accurately to observe the progress of the infection, I selected a healthy boy, about eight years old, for the purpose of inoculation for the Cow Pox. The matter was taken from a sore on the hand of a dairymaid*, who was infected by her master's cows, and it was inserted, on the 14th of May, 1796, into the arm of the boy by means of two superficial incisions, barely penetrating the cutis, each about half an inch long.
>
> *From the sore on the hand of Sarah Nelmes.[11]

Jenner had performed the world's first "vaccination." The experimental vaccination of James Phipps separated Jenner from those who earlier had casually observed the power of cowpox to prevent smallpox. Jenner was testing whether the cowpox virus could be transmitted from one human being to another, *without any contact with an infected cow*, by means of inoculation (vaccination) and retain its capacity to prevent smallpox in the recipient.

Would James Phipps become infected with cowpox? Jenner followed the progress of his young patient (Case 17) with care. He describes the course of a mild illness that lasted from the seventh to the ninth day following vaccination. The symptoms included loss of appetite, a slight headache, and restlessness. It appeared as if Jenner's cowpox inoculation had indeed transmitted the disease of cowpox from Sarah Nelmes to James Phipps. But the question still remained: had the properties of *V. vaccinae* that protected against smallpox also been transmitted? Jenner's next step was to test James Phipps's susceptibility to smallpox:

> In order to ascertain whether the boy, after feeling so slight an affection of the system from the Cow-pox virus, was secure from the contagion of the Smallpox, he was inoculated [variolated] the 1st of July following with variolous matter, immediately taken from a [smallpox] pustule. Several slight punctures and incisions were made on both his arms, and the matter was carefully inserted, *but no disease followed.* . . . [12] Several months afterwards, he was again inoculated with variolous matter, but no sensible effect was produced on the constitution.

The Nelmes-Phipps experiment demonstrated that cowpox virus could be transmitted through a human being and retain its capacity to immunize against smallpox. The word used for this kind of transmission at the time was "passaged." The disease produced in James Phipps by vaccination with the cowpox matter taken from Sarah Nelmes had the same properties as the disease produced by direct contact with an infected cow. The original infective agent had not mutated into something else. This was Jenner's crucial finding.

Cowpox was a disease that was prevalent in relatively few regions of the world, and the successful transmission of the V. vaccinae from person to person, without loss of its essential properties, meant that protection against smallpox could be transmitted using human beings as the agents of transmission. Direct cow-to-person transmission was not necessary. The knowledge that an infected cow was needed only as an initial source of the cowpox virus made it possible to envision vaccination as a universal solution to smallpox. Jenner immediately recognized the potential of his discovery, and the transmission of his cowpox vaccine began forthwith.

The purpose of the remaining experiments cited in the Inquiry—Cases 18 through 23—was to reproduce the results observed in the Nelmes-Phipps transmission. Jenner wanted to determine how long he could continue to produce effective immunity to smallpox by inoculating a chain of individuals with cowpox matter. But Jenner had to wait: in 1797 there were no cows infected with cowpox to be found in Gloucestershire:

> My researches were interrupted till the spring of the year 1798, when . . . the Cow-pox broke out among several of our dairies, which afforded me an opportunity of making further observations upon this curious disease.[13]

On March 16, 1798, Jenner initiated a series of cowpox inoculations beginning with William Summers, age five, whom he inoculated with lymph obtained directly from an infected cow.[14] Twelve days later (March 28) he took liquid matter from the vaccination lesion on the arm of William Summers and inoculated William Pead, age eight.[15] Eight days later (April 5) he used the Summers virus again to inoculate several more children and a few adults.[16] Jenner seems to have been testing just how long cowpox virus could remain viable and capable of infecting new recipients. From among the children inoculated on April 5, Jenner chose Hannah Excell, a seven-year-old girl; on April 12 he used matter taken from the pock on her arm to inoculate four other children between the ages of eleven months and six years.[17] Of these children, Mary Pead, age five, provided cowpox lymph to inoculate J. Barge, a boy of seven, the twenty-third and final case in the series.[18]

Surprisingly, given Jenner's fastidious documentation of personal names and vaccination dates, in the case of the Barge child he mentions neither the child's full name nor the date of his vaccination, but he is unlikely to have inoculated the Barge boy before April 17. Several days would have been required for the children who were inoculated on April 12 to develop pocks with sufficient cowpox lymph to vaccinate other children. Jenner normally waited seven or eight days between inoculations; therefore, a reasonable estimated date for the vaccination of J. Barge is April 20, or later.

Jenner left for London on April 24, which means that he did not have time to follow the Barge child closely or to test the boy's reaction to variolation.[19] Having satisfied himself that he had sufficient evidence to demonstrate that inoculation with cowpox lymph (vaccination) would prevent smallpox, Jenner was eager to arrange for the publication of his results. He delegated the final cases to his nephew, Henry Jenner, and then included the younger man's report in the *Inquiry*:

> I [Henry Jenner] have inoculated [with smallpox] Pead and Barge, two of the boys whom you lately infected with the Cow-pox. . . . He [Barge] sickened on the 8th day, went through the disease [of smallpox] with the usual slight symptoms, and without any inflammation on the arm beyond the common efflorescence surrounding the pustule, an appearance so often seen in inoculated Smallpox. . . .[20]

Having concluded that the protective power of the cowpox virus could be transmitted from human to human, perhaps indefinitely, Jenner summarized his investigations into the "curious disease of cowpox" in a single paragraph:

> These experiments afforded me much satisfaction, they proved that the [cowpox] matter in passing from one human subject to another, through five gradations, lost none of its original properties, J. Barge being the fifth who received the infection successively from William Summers, the boy to whom it was communicated from the cow.[21]

Jenner ended his *Inquiry* with a discursive essay that offered an interpretation of his findings and speculation about their implications. Acknowledging that he was not the first to observe that individuals who had been infected with cowpox failed to get smallpox, Jenner's more general observations set him apart from previous observers. He engaged his reader in a thoughtful discussion of the broad range of considerations that informed his investigations and conclusions.

Jenner the Naturalist theorized about the origins of cowpox: the infection, he thought, was transmitted from the horse to the cow by farmhands who handled both animals. Jenner the Epidemiologist considered the importance of environmental and social factors in the distribution and dissemination of this disease. Why, he asked, was cowpox a disease unknown in Ireland? Because, he suggested, in Ireland, only men worked with horses and only women milked cows; therefore, opportunities to transmit the virus from the horse to the cow did not exist in Ireland.

Jenner the Physician informed his colleagues that cowpox, unlike smallpox, was not contagious. It cannot, he insisted, be passed casually from one person to another: the children he had inoculated with cowpox did not even infect the siblings with whom they shared beds. Finally, Jenner the Realist offered practical advice on how to improve the practice of variolation to reduce the mortality caused by it: "barely scratch the surface of the skin," he wrote. He knew that it would be many years before cowpox inoculation (vaccination) could replace variolation and eradicate the universal threat of smallpox.

But Jenner left no doubt about his conviction that, in time, inoculation with cowpox virus would prove far superior to even the most cautiously administered variolation:

> Should it be asked whether this investigation is a matter of mere curiosity, or whether it tends to any beneficial purpose? I should answer, that notwithstanding the happy effects of Inoculation [variolation], with all the improvements which the practice has received since its first introduction into this country, it not very infrequently produces deformity of the skin, and sometimes, under the best management, proves fatal.[22]

Jenner the Scientist concluded his inquiry with a challenge to his colleagues to test and verify his findings and a promise to continue his own research:

> Thus far have I proceeded in an inquiry, founded, as it must appear, on the basis of experiment; in which, however, conjecture has been occasionally admitted in order to present to persons well situated for such discussions, objects for a more minute investigation. In the mean time I shall myself continue to prosecute this inquiry, encouraged by the hope of its becoming essentially beneficial to mankind.[23]

Two centuries later, Edward Jenner's experiments and his understanding of their implications still seem remarkable. That he proceeded from theory to experiment was not unusual at the time. Nor was it unusual that he engaged in clinical trials and published his results. His fascination with comparative anatomy and the physiology of different species, his surgical training, and his extensive collaboration with John Hunter predisposed Jenner to his approach to puzzling questions. This kind of scientific investigation was fairly standard among natural historians and clinical investigators.

But Jenner's cowpox experiments required more than clinical training and a scientific outlook. They required the active collaboration of local inhabitants. Jenner's experiments involved infecting the children of local families with a nasty bovine disease. Why did they allow it? He clearly had their trust, but it was not a blind trust. Jenner's knowledge would not have been unfamiliar to the farming families of the children he inoculated. They would have known that cowpox broke out in local herds from time to time, that occasionally it infected the people who handled the cows, and that cowpox was not a serious, life-threatening disease. Like Jenner they may also have been acquainted with the local folk wisdom that people who had been infected with cowpox did not get smallpox.

They would also have known that variolation, which had been practiced in England for more than half a century, was extremely risky. They knew that the purpose of variolation was to produce a mild case of smallpox, but they also knew it could provoke a serious or even fatal case. The notion that purposeful inoculation with cowpox virus might protect their children against smallpox must have had a certain appeal. With exposure to natural smallpox a virtual certainty, they had little to lose by letting Jenner try his experiment. It just might work.

While the concept of "informed consent" as we know it today did not exist, there can be little doubt that the children's parents were "informed" participants in Jenner's experiments. Jenner had both a persuasive argument and an informed constituency. In fact, Jenner must have had not only their consent but their active collaboration. His busy practice covered a large rural area, and he would have had to depend on reports of family members to track the course of the disease of cowpox in those he inoculated. Jenner's status as country doctor was an asset in both a scientific and a social sense: the task he set himself was to track the transmission of an infectious disease from farm animals to human subjects. This required being close to the scene and having a familiar and knowledgeable population with which to work.

Fear may have been Jenner's most important ally. Eighteenth-century parents had to accept the inevitability of smallpox. They knew its terrible toll: one child in four would die of the disease, and those who recovered were likely to be blind or disfigured for life. The known options with which to combat this certainty were both limited and risky: parents could hope for the best while waiting for natural smallpox to strike, or they could have their children inoculated with smallpox matter. Jenner presented a third option: allow me inoculate your child with cowpox matter. A mild illness of short duration will follow, after which I will inoculate him or her with smallpox. If successful, your child will no longer have to fear exposure to smallpox, and we will learn whether inoculation with cowpox can prevent smallpox. Families that permitted Jenner to vaccinate their children had no reason to believe that they were taking a great risk with their lives or their health. The knowledge they shared with their physician was powerful and persuasive.

DIFFUSION

Unlike the diffusion of knowledge about variolation, which took more than a century, the diffusion of information about Jenner's cowpox experiments was exceedingly rapid. Diffusion began with the publication of Jenner's *Inquiry* in London in midsummer 1798. Jenner's treatise was not entirely unknown at the time: a few friends and colleagues in Gloucestershire and other parts of England had read and commented on early drafts.

Jenner anticipated that his *Inquiry* would be read by his British medical colleagues, and that they would repeat and verify his findings. Prominent London physicians, and less prominent physicians elsewhere, began immediately to test Jenner's claims. Richard Dunning, a Plymouth physician, quickly coined the term "vaccination" (derived from Jenner's *vaccinae*) in *Some Observations on Vaccination*, a pamphlet published in London in 1800.[24] The term caught on, but "cowpox inoculation" and "inoculating the cow pox" were used as well, causing some confusion, because variolation was also called "inoculation." Interested physicians became participants in the dissemination of information: they published articles about their results and sent queries to the medical journals of the day to learn what others had found. Dunning, who became an active supporter of Jenner, sent queries to the *Medical and Physical Journal* designed to elicit public answers from Jenner. The turnaround was rapid: in one instance, a question raised in the issue of May 1800 received a prompt reply from Jenner in the June issue.[25]

One problem with testing Jenner's results was the continuing difficulty in finding cows infected with cowpox. George Pearson of St. Luke's Hospital and William Woodville of London's Smallpox and Inoculation Hospital found infected cows in dairy herds near London about six months after the publication of Jenner's treatise, but Pearson had published his thoughts on vaccination even before he had an opportunity to witness the cowpox method personally.[26] Pearson was sufficiently convinced of the veracity of Jenner's claim to open a subscription to support a London clinic where the poor could bring their children to be vaccinated without charge. The clinic opened for business on December 2, 1798, with a physician and surgeon in attendance.[27]

By the spring of 1799, Woodville had vaccinated more than 500 individuals in the London Smallpox Hospital and published his results as *Reports of a Series of Inoculations for the Variolae Vaccinae or Cow-Pox*.[28] Woodville confirmed Jenner's findings. He and Pearson were among the first to experiment with cowpox inoculation, and although both would later become sharp critics of Jenner, initially they were strong supporters and an early source of information about vaccination in the British Isles.[29]

Knowledge of Jenner's discovery moved rapidly beyond Britain. Although Britain and France were at war and Napoleon's advances dominated life in Europe during the early years of the nineteenth century, news about vaccination spread almost immediately to the continent. Well-developed medical and scientific networks connected Britain to the countries of Western Europe, as well as to the seaboard communities of North America. This "western" medical network consisted of physicians who had studied medicine in Britain, France, the Netherlands, Austria, and Germany. Many were members of the same medical and scientific societies. If they did not know each other personally, they might be acquainted through their publications in European and British medical books and journals. Articles and books of general interest to the medical community were translated with amazing speed into the various European languages early in the nineteenth century. Although the contingencies of war may have slowed or shifted the normal channels through which information traveled, places with even tenuous connections to European nations had soon heard about vaccination.

A large number of European immigrants who had fled the upheavals in Europe were resident in Britain when Edward Jenner published his *Inquiry*, and their presence helped speed the diffusion process. The Swiss—especially Genevans—played an important role in the early transmission to the continent of knowledge about vaccination. The *Bibliothèque britannique,* a relatively new monthly publication founded in Geneva in 1796, made current English-language literature available to the French-reading public of Europe. Marc-Auguste Pictet, a professor at the University of Geneva, was in London in September 1798 to collect material for the next issue, and he returned to Geneva with a copy of Jenner's *Inquiry.* The first announcement of Jenner's discovery in Europe appeared in the October issue of the *Bibliothèque britannique*:

> Dr. Edward Jenner of Berkeley in Gloucestershire has demonstrated by a multitude of carefully performed observations and tests that all those who have had this illness [cowpox] are forever protected from ordinary smallpox and made incapable of contracting it, either by contagion or inoculations.[30]

Bibliothèque britannique became a virtual propaganda sheet for vaccination in Napoleon's expanding French empire and in France itself. The November and December issues carried an almost complete French translation of Jenner's *Inquiry.* Dr. Louis Odier, the translator, was a physician and native of Geneva who had been educated at the University of Edinburgh. Other European language translations of *Inquiry* appeared quickly. Aloysio Careno, an Italian physician, published a Latin edition in 1799, and a German translation by G. Fr. Ballhorn was published in Hanover the same year. French and Italian translations were published in 1800 in Lyon and Pavia, respectively. The first Dutch edition was translated and published in Haarlem in 1801 by Leonardus Davids, a Rotterdam physician and early supporter of Edward Jenner. Table 2.1 shows the years and languages in which the earliest editions of Jenner's *Inquiry* were published.

The continuing conversations between Jenner and his many friends and colleagues in the years following the publication of *Inquiry* eventually connected individuals in many parts of the world. Until his death in 1823, Jenner himself responded to a host of questions, reports, and comments opposed to infecting children with the cowpox virus. He also corresponded with a widening range of physicians who reported their own results with vaccination to him personally. *V. vaccinae*'s passage across the North Atlantic occurred quickly and easily. In 1798, Jenner sent a copy of his *Inquiry* and a sample of cowpox lymph to John Clinch, one of his earliest friends and a doctor and

TABLE 2.1

Early editions and translations of Edward Jenner's Inquiry

Year	Place	Language	Edition
1798	London	English	First
1799	Vienna	Latin	First
	Hanover	German	First
1800	London	English	Second
	Lyon	French	First
	Pavia	Italian	First
1801	London	English	Third
	Haarlem	Dutch	First
	Madrid	Spanish	First
1802	Springfield	English	First
	Massachusetts		American
1803	Lisbon	Portuguese	First

SOURCE: W. R. LeFanu, *A Bio-bibliography of Edward Jenner, 1749-1823* (Philadelphia: J. B. Lippincott Company, 1951), 38-43. Jenner's biographer, John Baron, in *The Life of Edward Jenner*, claimed that a Spanish translation was published in Madrid in 1801 (London: H. Colburn, 1827-1838), 393. LeFanu (1951) states that no Spanish translation for that year has been found.

clergyman in Newfoundland, and Clinch became the Western Hemisphere's first vaccinator.

Jenner also sent cowpox lymph to Benjamin Waterhouse, a Boston physician who had met Jenner while studying medicine in Britain. Waterhouse had spent seven years studying in London, Edinburgh, and Leiden, and was perhaps the best-educated physician in North America. In 1800, Waterhouse vaccinated his four children and two servants and then exposed them to smallpox without ill effect.[31] He actively promoted the use of vaccination in North America throughout his life, and he introduced Thomas Jefferson to the procedure. Jefferson would become one of the most active supporters of vaccination in the United States. With this kind of elite patronage, vaccination gained an early and strong foothold in the eastern United States where population was sparse, smallpox epidemics less frequent, and the disease more likely to kill both adults and children. The rapid diffusion of information about this new medical technique demonstrates the degree to which personal, political, and professional networks connected the Western world in the early nineteenth century—a transatlantic Western world that included the Atlantic seaboard of the newly created United States.

The early and successful transmission of live cowpox virus from England to North America might lead one to conclude that the dissemination of vaccine depended upon little more than a connection between acquaintances, the delivery of a small amount of live cowpox lymph, and an interested recipient. Nothing could be further from the truth. The easy passage across the North Atlantic was deceptive: *V. vaccinae* survived best and longest in cool climates. However effortlessly and quickly the cowpox virus was transmitted to North America, its survival depended on human assistance. Unlike the smallpox virus, which could be found just about anywhere in the world, the cowpox virus had to be transported from western Europe to the rest of the world. The transmission of Jenner's cowpox vaccine to warmer climes and across greater distances would require extraordinary commitment, ingenuity, and perseverance.

Jenner was well aware of the problems of preserving the vitality of the cowpox virus. When writing to Jean de Carro in Vienna in November 1799, Jenner described the technique he used to preserve the virus:

> I have enclos'd two portions of the Virus taken from different subjects: & with the view of excluding Oxygen as much as possible, I have plac'd it between two pieces of Glass. The quantity is larger than it appears, as so much evaporation takes place in drying. When you make use of it, moisten it either by taking up a very small portion of water on the point of your Lancet, or by breathing upon it.[32]

Jean de Carro was another displaced physician from Geneva with a medical degree from Edinburgh who had moved to Vienna after Napoleon's rise to power in France. When he wrote to Jenner on September 14, 1800, he had already received live cowpox virus from another source. He wrote to report his success with vaccination and to request fresh lymph.[33] Jenner was delighted: "I cannot forbear congratulating you on the success you have already met with, although it must be confess'd that congratulation bears hard upon egotism."[34]

This exchange was the beginning of a ten-year correspondence between Jenner, De Carro, and Alexandre J. G. Marcet, another physician from Geneva who had been educated at Edinburgh, which partially documents the early migration of the cowpox virus eastward.[35] Initially transmission of the virus was from place to place and person to person within the British foreign diplomatic establishment. De Carro, for example, supplied cowpox lymph to Lord and Lady Elgin, who were on their way to Constantinople to visit their daughter. The Elgins passed it on to the British Consul at Saloniki, who in turn sent it to Hartford Jones, the British Resident in Baghdad. Precisely how the virus was conveyed in all these instances is not known, but variations on Jenner's suggested method of conveyance seem to have prevailed. In the last of these transmissions the virus was placed on a piece of linen, sealed between two plates of glass, and sealed again within a wax ball. By July 1802, *V. vaccinae* had traveled from London to Bombay.

Direct transmission of cowpox across the English Channel to France proved more difficult for different reasons. When Jenner published his treatise, Britain and France were at war and communications between the two countries were irregular. Even so, information about vaccination reached France quickly via personal and professional connections. In 1799, the French Society of Medicine in Paris published a review of *Inquiry* in the August-September issue of the Society's journal. Count Joseph de la Roque, a French *émigré* living in London, translated the first complete French edition of Jenner's treatise and published it in Lyon during the winter of 1799–1800. By the end of 1800, three subsequent French editions of Jenner's *Inquiry* had been published, and Antoine Aubert, a young Genevan doctor living in London, had published a French translation of Woodville's published reports on vaccination.[36]

The French Society of Medicine decided to initiate a formal investigation into the matter of vaccination and chose a celebrated psychiatrist, Philippe Pinel, to repeat Jenner's experiments and issue a report, but first he had to obtain the cowpox virus. Antoine Aubert returned to France with cowpox lymph he had obtained from Woodville, and he and Pinel inoculated three foundling children. Unfortunately, the virus had been taken from English patients who had been vaccinated more than two months earlier, the virus had lost its vitality, and the vaccinations failed. Aubert returned to England to consult with both Jenner and Woodville, and the latter allowed him to observe and vaccinate patients at the London Smallpox Hospital. Convinced that Jenner's claim was justified, Aubert sent more vaccine to Pinel, whose second attempt at vaccination on April 14, 1800, also failed.[37]

In the case of France, it was neither distance nor climate that slowed attempts to transfer cowpox from England to France, but the hostilities between the two countries. When it became clear that private initiatives were not working, vaccination advocates sought the assistance of the French government. Surprisingly, perhaps, it was not difficult to obtain. When Napoleon Bonaparte became dictator of France in November 1800, he permitted some exiled French *émigrés* to return to France. Among those who did so was La Rochefoucauld-Liancourt, an Enlightenment enthusiast who was living in

London when Jenner's treatise was published. La Rochefoucould knew about George Pearson's London Vaccination Institute, and he proposed founding a similar institution in Paris.[38] He had no difficulty attracting donations from some of the most distinguished doctors in Paris. Among the nonmedical subscribers were Napoleon's brother, Lucien Bonaparte, Minister of the Interior; and Charles Maurice Talleyrand, Minister of Foreign Affairs. The subscription was filled almost immediately.[39]

Preparations to test the vaccine continued. On May 11, 1800, subscribers met at the Medical School of the University of Paris to establish the institutional and operational machinery to begin experiments as soon as live cowpox virus became available.[40] A Central Committee of Vaccination was charged with verifying the English doctors' results and keeping detailed records of the findings. Nine doctors would perform the vaccinations, and an administrative committee of five would handle business matters and publicize the progress of the Committee's work in newspapers and journals.

With detailed bureaucratic procedures now in place, the Central Committee of Vaccination still had no vaccine, and Foreign Minister Talleyrand was approached for assistance. While Napoleon was crossing the Alps on his way to the battle of Marengo, Louis-Guillaume Otto, France's representative to England, was in London requesting vaccine from Pearson's London Vaccination Institute. Otto sent vaccine on May 27 that was used to vaccinate thirty French children on June 2, but despite the rapid transfer, this third attempt also failed.

At this point England's most experienced vaccinator, William Woodville, decided to go to France himself to assist the Central Committee. Talleyrand approved a passport for Woodville to enter France, but he was detained by the French authorities in Boulougne. While waiting for permission to proceed to Paris, Woodville vaccinated several children in Boulougne. He arrived in Paris on July 25, 1800, and vaccinated several children there without success, but he then learned that the unplanned vaccinations he had performed in Boulougne were successful. It was this Boulougne strain that established a source of V. *vaccinae* in France. In less than twenty-four hours, Woodville had vaccinated the eleven-month-old son of François Colon in Paris using lymph taken from a child vaccinated in Boulougne. This was an excellent tactical move. A public health officer, Colon was already promoting Jennerian vaccination, and in addition to offering his son as the repository of France's second generation of cowpox virus, he also offered his house on the Rue de Vaugirard to be used as a vaccination hospital.[41]

Vaccination spread throughout France with seemingly little resistance from French practitioners of variolation. With cowpox vaccine finally in hand, the Central Committee of Vaccination could proceed with its own investigations of Jenner's claim. Unlike in Britain, close collaboration between university physicians and the French government meant that France developed a systematic national program of clinical research and documentation, which helped enhance the reputation of vaccination in Europe. The Committee took a multipronged approach: devise ways to preserve the vaccine, develop plans to distribute vaccine to the prefectures of France, train physicians to perform vaccination, and publicize the benefits of vaccination. France began a three-year program of testing, but in October 1800, after 150 French children had been vaccinated, the Committee issued a preliminary report. The report strongly supported Jenner's claim: "All of those vaccinated have had the disease [of cowpox] very mildly; no accident has occurred."[42] Nor had any of the children subsequently variolated with the smallpox virus become infected with smallpox. In 1803 the Central Committee of Vaccination issued its final report: Jenner was correct, cowpox vaccination did prevent smallpox.

Despite the ingenuity of private individuals and the assistance of the French government, the need for permission to cross enemy lines significantly delayed the arrival of the cowpox virus. The vaccine reached France more than a year after it reached Switzerland and Austria. It was an early sign that international politics would impede the global distribution of cowpox vaccine. Impediments increased significantly as efforts to export this new medical technology reached beyond the contiguous European states. The extreme fragility of the cowpox virus was immediately recognized by those who tried to give or send it to others, and difficulties in maintaining the vitality of the virus remained the primary obstacle to the dissemination of vaccination for most of the nineteenth century. This fundamental challenge—keeping the required cowpox virus alive—was compounded by distance, as well as by political, institutional, environmental, and cultural barriers.

Despite these unalterable difficulties, live cowpox virus was transported and vaccination was introduced to all major world regions within a decade. However, conveying live virus beyond well-established European networks required much greater dedication and investment of resources. And as *V. vaccinae* traveled through diplomatic, military, and bureaucratic channels, more often than not, introducing vaccination required some measure of coercion.

The European powers that administered distant colonial empires had enormous incentives to promote methods of smallpox control in their colonies. In Spanish America and the British and Dutch East Indies, where population densities were high, smallpox was a constant threat to ruler and ruled alike. And in Australia, where the population was sparse and scattered, the demographic consequences of imported smallpox were horrifying. Smallpox mortality rates in rarely exposed populations could exceed 50 percent.

Colonial governments were in a position to impose vaccination on their subjects, and initially, at least, that is what they did. On the other hand, the colonial powers soon learned that the cooperation of local doctors was required over the longer term. The powerful demonstration effect of vaccination was especially helpful in this regard. When children who had not been vaccinated got smallpox and those who had been vaccinated did not, vaccination's case was made. But this took time, and before any such demonstration effect could begin, the European powers had to provide their distant colonial governments with cowpox vaccine.

Spain was among the first of the European powers to act decisively to introduce vaccination to its colonial empire.[43] And it was Spain that demonstrated the effectiveness of using children to convey live cowpox virus over long distances.

Knowledge of Jenner's discovery and cowpox vaccine reached Spain without difficulty. In January 1800, the *Gaceta de Madrid* reported that the Italian physician Careno had sent the Spanish king, Carlos IV, a copy of Jenner's treatise and linen threads impregnated with cowpox lymph.[44] The king's physician, Dr. José Felipe de Flores, declared smallpox to be the "first and principal cause of the depopulation of America,"[45] and the Spanish Council of the Indies considered control of this scourge to be an important state responsibility. In addition, Spain's colonial governments soon were clamoring for the Spanish government to send them vaccine. In June 1802, the Ayuntamiento of Santa Fé de Bogotá asked the king to send vaccine lymph to help control an epidemic of smallpox that had broken out that year.[46] Later the same year several issues of the *Gaceta de Guatemala* published vaccination instructions and reports about the cowpox method, simultaneously expressing frustration about the inability to get vaccine lymph from Spain.[47]

Early in 1803, Dr. José Felipé de Flores presented a report to the Council of the Indies in Madrid, recommending the dispatch of a royal expedition led by the most learned doctors from the Medical School of Cádiz. De Flores had successfully introduced variolation to Guatamala during a smallpox epidemic in 1780. He recommended that two ships be outfitted to transport cows infected with cowpox, a quantity of cowpox vaccine sealed between glass slides, and a sufficient number of nonimmune young boys to allow successive vaccination during the trip. One or a combination of these methods, it was hoped, would insure the safe arrival of live cowpox virus in the New World. One ship would go to New Spain via Havana, Puerto Rico, Guatemala, and the Yucatán; the second would go to Cartagena to dispatch lymph to Santa Fé de Bogatá, Guayra, Montevideo, Portobello, Panama, and other southern dominions. The vaccine was to be distributed to major cities, where the government, principal citizens, and selected Spanish physicians would supervise the preservation and propagation of the vaccine virus. Vaccine would then be dispatched to the provincial capitals and municipalities, which would adopt a similar procedure and distribute vaccine to villages within their jurisdiction.

The scope and details of this plan suggest that the characteristics of the cowpox virus were well understood and that communications between the Spanish government and Central and South America were excellent. To insure compliance in the Spanish colonies, the Catholic Church would play a major role. When an infant was baptized, the priest would require the godparents to return within six months to have the child vaccinated, offer an indulgence authorized by the Pope, and have a physician or priest record the child's vaccination in a special parish registry. Bishops would inspect parish records during diocesan visits, and other colonial officials would encourage the acceptance of vaccination by both example and decree. Each Audiencia would require priests to submit an annual report on the progress of immunization in each parish, which the Audiencia could then report to the king.[48]

This was a plan on a grand scale. De Flores's proposal envisioned surveillance from the top to be supported by all levels of the bureaucracy. Reports were to flow from the bottom up. The plan indicates a clear understanding of the need to establish a local supply of vaccine in the Spanish colonies once lymph had been introduced from Europe. This reality could be achieved only by vaccinating the children of the resident population, a policy that was likely to be resisted and that would require the full support of the colonial authorities. De Flores also recognized the need for systematic documentation of the successes and failures of the government's vaccination program.

The Spanish government responded quickly to De Flores's proposal. On March 3, 1803, Carlos IV ordered the Council to report on the possibility of sending cowpox lymph to Spanish colonies.[49] On March 22, the Council approved De Flores's recommendations and proposed that a physician and some young boys from La Casa de Desamparados, a foundling home in Madrid, accompany the regular packet ship to Veracruz. De Flores himself would go to Veracruz to direct lymph to Peru, Costa Rica, Nicaragua, and Guatemala via Cumaná, Caracas, and Cartagena. The physician Francisco Xavier de Balmis y Berenguer would command the Mexican expedition.[50] Balmis, a resident of New Spain for many years, recently had translated a French treatise on vaccination entitled *Tratado histórico y practicó de la vacuna*. When the vaccine reached Mexico, the viceroy and provincial governors were to supervise the propagation of the virus by vaccinating children throughout the colony. In May 1803, the king approved a "Real Expedición Marítima de la Vacuna" to the New World.

A majority of the Council members recommended that the Royal Treasury bear the initial expenses; reimbursement from municipal funds from the towns that benefited could come later. The Governor of the Council of the Indies, the Marqués de Bajamar, dissented. He argued that the loss of life from smallpox in the colonies was so enormous that the Royal Treasury should absorb all the costs of the expedition, because the long-term economic benefits would more than repay the investment. The king approved Bajamar's recommendation: in early June, he instructed the Junta de Cirujanos de Cámara (Council of Chamber Surgeons) to select three physicians to direct separate expeditions to Buenos Aires, Mexico, and Lima; determine the salaries and funds needed; and organize the expedition. Each physician was to choose boys from the Casa de Niños Espósitos and the Casa de Desamparados in Madrid. The children would remain in the care of the colonial viceroys until they reached legal age or found a suitable position. The Spanish physicians would teach local practitioners how to vaccinate and distribute cowpox vaccine to the provincial capitals and principal cities of each viceroyalty. The royal order was intended to impress the viceroys with the importance of the mission and encourage the bishops and other clergy to support it.

Dr. Francisco Xavier de Balmis was appointed to serve as director of the expedition to New Spain in June 1803. To insure unmolested passage, he solicited passes of safe conduct from the belligerents in the Napoleonic Wars, and what became known as the Balmis Expedition was underway by the end of the year. Balmis sailed from La Coruña in the *María Pita* on November 30, 1803, with a "director, three assistants, two practitioners, three male nurses, a secretary, the ex-rectores, and twenty-two young boys who had not had smallpox."[51] The twenty-two boys were deemed a sufficient number to transmit the cowpox vaccine during the transatlantic voyage. The ages of the boys ranged from three to nine years. Two of them were to be vaccinated every ninth or tenth day. If one boy destroyed his vaccination vesicle, or it otherwise became ineffective, the second boy's remained available for subsequent vaccinations. To quote Michael Smith, "these twenty-two innocents formed the most vital element of the most ambitious medical enterprise any government had ever undertaken."[52] The transmission strategy worked: Jenner's cowpox vaccine was transported from Spain to Central and South America using the same arm-to-arm transmission method that Jenner had used to conduct his vaccination experiments in Gloucestershire five years earlier.

Not satisfied with the transatlantic transmission of the cowpox virus to the Spanish colonies in the Americas, in March 1805, Francisco Xavier de Balmis set sail for the Philippine Islands. He chose twenty-six Mexican boys to accompany him on the long voyage.[53] Balmis complained about the cramped conditions aboard ship, which required the boys to sleep next to one another and caused unplanned, premature vaccinations. He reported that the number of carriers would not have been sufficient to preserve the virus had not favorable winds brought them into port ahead of schedule.[54] He arrived in Manila on April 15 after a five-week journey, and began to vaccinate children the following day. When the Royal Expedition returned to New Spain fourteen months later, 20,000 islanders had been vaccinated.[55]

In late summer, Balmis moved on to the Portuguese colony at Macao. He took with him three Philippino boys whose services had been volunteered by a priest at the Church of Santa Cruz. After a pleasant eight-day voyage, they encountered a typhoon on September 10 as they sailed into Macao harbor. The storm prevented them from landing for another six days, but despite this unexpected delay, the vaccine survived. Balmis was welcomed by the agents of the Royal Philippine Company who enthusiastically encouraged vaccination in Macao. Balmis's welcome may have been due in part to the fact that the benefits of vaccination were already known in Macao. Don Pedro Huet, a Portuguese subject and merchant of Macao, had brought cowpox vaccine to Macao from the Philippines on the *Esperanza* four months earlier, and for a short period, vaccination had been practiced by the Portuguese physicians there.[56] However, the vitality of the virus had not been properly maintained, and the Portuguese welcomed its reintroduction. Balmis stayed in Macao for a few weeks to train local physicians in the techniques necessary to transmit and preserve the virus.

Intending to introduce the vaccine virus in China, Balmis and a single youth sailed for Canton on October 5, 1805. Balmis spoke no Chinese and needed an intermediary, but he was not welcomed in this port city. The Spanish-speaking agents of the Royal Philippine Company in Canton showed little interest in Balmis's mission and refused to seek the cooperation of the Chinese officials. Balmis was reduced to paying small amounts to poor families living along the Pearl River to allow him to vaccinate their children simply to keep the virus alive. He then turned to agents of the British East India Company, who welcomed him and his vaccine. News of vaccination had reached Canton in 1803 and vaccine had been sent from Bombay and other parts of British-controlled territories in Asia that year, but when the vaccine arrived, the virus was no longer viable.[57]

With the transfer of live vaccine to knowledgeable British authorities in Canton, Balmis had accomplished his goal of introducing vaccination to China. Alexander Pearson, the Senior Surgeon at the British East India Company in Canton, was familiar with vaccination, and he had written a tract explaining its benefits and how to do the procedure. His *Treatise on the European Style of Vaccination* was translated into Chinese by Sir George Thomas Stanton, an English resident in Canton, and Cheng Ch'ung-ch'ien, and published as *Ying-ch'i-li kuo hsin ch'u chung tou ch'i shu (Novel Book on the New Method of Inoculation, Lately Out of England)* in 1805.[58] The East India Company opened a public vaccination clinic in December and hired a full-time physician to administer the vaccine.[59] Vaccination did not immediately gain the support of Chinese physicians in South China, where Chinese-style variolation was a widely used and accepted medical technique; however, when a smallpox epidemic struck Canton in the winter of 1805–1806, many Chinese brought their children to the clinic to be vaccinated. Vaccination and variolation would co-exist in China: both techniques were effective, and both had committed advocates in the medical profession.

Francisco Xavier de Balmis had extended his efforts on behalf of vaccination well beyond the Spanish sphere of influence. Having transported the cowpox virus from Cádiz to Canton, he returned to Macao to begin the long voyage home to Spain. He was received personally by King Carlos IV and accorded a hero's welcome on September 7, 1806.[60]

While *V. vaccinae* made its way eastward through British diplomatic and professional channels, and westward under the auspices of the Spanish empire, it was being conveyed in a much less predictable fashion by a great assortment of individuals acting on their own initiative. Individuals who believed that vaccination could prevent smallpox, and had by some means acquired cowpox lymph, simply acted on this belief when an opportunity to introduce the virus presented itself. Unlike the reports routinely sent to the Spanish government, the successes and failures of these independent initiatives were reported, if at all, in personal correspondence, in newspaper articles, in popular and scientific journals, and by word of mouth. Some of these reports have survived, and they provide a patchwork of information that reveals, at least in part, important routes of transmission taken by Jenner's cowpox vaccine.

Dissemination of the vaccine to the countries of Southeast Asia required contact and cooperation among the French, English, and Dutch colonial governments that were at war in the early 1800s. At that time, Île de France (Mauritius) and Réunion in the Indian Ocean were administered by France;[61] and the island of Java in Indonesia, with its capital at Batavia (Jakarta), was held by the Dutch. Napoleon Bonaparte had conquered the Republic of the Netherlands in 1794–95 and the Dutch were bound to France by alliance.[62] French control did not extend to the Dutch colonies in the Netherlands East Indies, but the British blockade of both France and Holland had virtually cut the Dutch East Indies off from the mother country.

Vaccination had attracted strong support from physicians in Holland, but Dutch ships were unable to send cowpox virus to Batavia. Instead, French colonial physicians and officials arranged to send vaccine lymph to the Dutch in Batavia, requiring collaboration between these two warring governments. A letter reporting the details of this transmission was sent by a physician on the Île de France to the editor of the *Philadelphia Medical and Physical Journal* and published in 1806.[63]

The physician was M. Laborde, head of medical services for the French islands of Île de France and Réunion in the late eighteenth and early nineteenth centuries. In 1792, he had witnessed a smallpox epidemic that had killed one-quarter of the islands' populations, and when he learned about Jenner's cowpox method, he was eager to try it. Laborde seems to have had excellent connections to sources of information about vaccination in England, France, and the United States. The events described in his letter took place sometime in 1803:

Dear Sir,

You requested me to send to you, before my departure from New-York, an account of the introduction and of the success of Vaccination, in the Isles of France and Réunion.

As soon as I heard of the discovery of Jenner, the experiments of Woodville, &c., I wrote to the latter; I invited him to become the benefactor of the colony. I also wrote to France. The war rendered communications difficult. At length, a French captain, coming from India, had the good fortune to preserve the virus fresh, by successive vaccinations made from arm to arm, during the voyage. He had also brought impregnated threads. I made a completely successful use of both sources, in the Hospital of the State. It was from these vaccinations, that I was enabled to furnish virus to the medical practitioners of the colony.

The transmission was equally successful in every quarter. Its operation was visible between the 4th and 5th day; and it was always from the commencement of the 8th to the close of the 9th day, that the virus in the pustule was of a clearness, and gumminess fit for transmission.

We have known of no adverse case in this practice, which has become general in the Isles of France and Réunion. It has been tried upon persons of every age; upon infants, from the 5th day after birth; upon pregnant females, without any preparation, or subsequent medical treatment; and the effect of the operation has, in almost every instance, been so light as scarcely to prove an inconvenience. ...There are some few examples of a more violent effect, and two or three of convulsions: *but not one of its ever proving mortal. . . .* I believe I am correct in saying, that, except those recently born, and those who daily arrive, *there is not, in the Isles of France and Réunion, a single individual who had not had the small-pox, that has not been vaccinated.*[64]

The threat of "those who daily arrive," however, remained a problem, and Laborde turned his attention to vaccinating the passengers on the ships that arrived with cases of smallpox on board. His letter to the *Philadelphia Medical and Physical Journal* documents the serious nature of smallpox on sailing vessels in the early nineteenth century, as well as the degree of coercion that could be, and was, applied to subject populations by colonial governments and by the captains of seafaring vessels:

A ship stored with Negroes arrived at the Island, with the small-pox on board. Fifteen or eighteen persons, had already died of it: a like number was, at the moment, under the effects of the confluent sort, and the number every day increased.[65] It was impossible to admit this vessel, both on account of the number of persons, who, at this time, had not been vaccinated, as well as on account of the then want of confidence in the protecting power of vaccination. It was necessary, therefore, to make the ship perform a quarantine at one of the Schychelles.

I placed on board six children of those first vaccinated. I directed the surgeon (whom I had placed on board the vessel for this purpose) to keep these children constantly among those who were infected with the small-pox: to make them eat and drink out of the same plates and cups; to make them wear the linen of the sick; and, finally, to inoculate them frequently with variolous matter. I likewise caused to be taken on board, a child, that had been vaccinated, and the matter of whose pustule was in the proper state for communication, in order to vaccinate forty of the negroes who had not then taken sick.

The result of these trials was, that the six vaccinated children were completely preserved, and that the success which attended the vaccination of the blacks was so perfect, that the small-pox became extinct. These were no more sick after the second day: many of them took the vaccine, and had the pustule.[66]

Laborde's primary goal may have been to prevent smallpox from reinfecting the island population for which he was responsible, but he had a multiple agenda. He was also conducting experiments on a transient population for which he was not responsible, and his tactics seem extreme: there was no question of consent among the captive Negro population, presumably slaves; nor is it likely that the parents of the six local children who were placed on board had much say in the matter. On the other hand, it is also clear, based on what Laborde had witnessed himself, that he had good reason to believe that vaccination would stop the spread of the smallpox epidemic on the ship, and that the local children he had already vaccinated would not contract smallpox. His experiment was based on his own experiences with vaccination and knowledge from sources he trusted.

Laborde ended his account much as Edward Jenner had ended his treatise— with a ringing endorsement of the cowpox method. His letter to the Philadelphia periodical was a testimonial intended to convince his medical colleagues in the United States to follow his example. As he described it, vaccination was an entirely benign procedure that could effectively eradicate smallpox everywhere:

I feel happy in believing that the knowledge of this fact [vaccination] (which is familiarly known to the whole Colony) will appear to you of a nature to subdue the most refractory unbelievers in the preserving power of the vaccine disorder. I know not the prevailing opinion relative to this practice in the

United-States; but I hope it will become universal; that quitting inoculation, which perpetuates the variolous infection, they will adopt VACCINATION, which destroys it.

> I remain, &c.
> LABORDE, D.M.
> New-York, August 29, 1805.[67]

Meanwhile, *V. vaccinae* had made its way from Île de France and Réunion to Batavia, the Dutch colonial capital on the island of Java in the Dutch East Indies. Sometime in late 1803, Lieutenant-General De Caen, Governor of the two French islands, sent the *Marengo*, a man-of-war, to Batavia with a sample of the virus and a letter describing the success the French were having with vaccination.[68] The virus did not survive the voyage, and Governor-General Siberg at Batavia wrote to De Caen to report that the vaccine was ineffective. He announced that he would soon send a ship to Île de France with a physician, Dr. Gauffre, and ten or twelve children who were to be vaccinated in turn on the return voyage. Siberg sent a letter to De Caen dated September 14, 1804, acknowledging that the vaccine had arrived in good condition and that children were being vaccinated successfully in Batavia.[69]

* * *

As these accounts attest, despite the problems associated with the global dissemination of Jenner's cowpox vaccine, live cowpox virus had been introduced to all regions of the world within five years after the publication of his *Inquiry*. It is important to remember that this global transmission depended entirely upon the availability and use of young children, frequently orphans who could be compelled to sail on long, difficult voyages, as carriers of *V. vaccinae*. It would not have been possible without them. The arm-to-arm method of vaccination would remain the favored mode of transmission—the only method that ensured a fresh supply of cowpox lymph—throughout the nineteenth century. When children were not available, the method Jenner had devised as an alternative—storing and conveying cowpox lymph in a glass tube or between two pieces of glass sealed with wax—was used. However, as will shortly become clear, these methods were not nearly as reliable.

Edward Jenner remained an active participant in the global web that promoted vaccination until his death in 1823. He maintained a voluminous correspondence with individuals throughout the world, dispensing encouragement and praise. Upon request, he would prepare and send cowpox lymph, with instructions on how to use it, to many correspondents he never met. And, not infrequently, he expressed great frustration toward the many who took a stand against vaccination. Jenner was directly involved in the transmission of cowpox vaccine to Europe, the Middle East, and North America, but did not participate in the diffusion of vaccination to Central or South America, or to Southeast and Eastern Asia. He functioned, however, as a central repository of information about the international progress of vaccination—information he then shared with friends and colleagues. Writing to John Addington, a London surgeon, in 1803:

> Allow me to congratulate you & and all lovers of the Vaccine, on the introduction of our little Pearl into India. This intelligence reach'd me yesterday from De Carro at Vienna & from a Gentleman just arrived from Madras.[70]

In a letter written on November 21, 1806, to Alexandre J. G. Marcet, another London colleague, Jenner could conceal neither his delight nor his chagrin over the remarkable success of Spain's Balmis Expedition:

> A few days since, I rec'd from Madrid a Document respecting Vaccination which fills me with more astonishment than anything that has yet reach'd me on that subject. It comes in the form of "Suplemento a la Gazeta [sic] de Madrid." I will get it printed and contrive to send you a copy. . . . Would to Heaven the British Cabinet had shewn the same Philanthropic Spirit as that of Spain![71]

And again, when he received a copy of Alexander Pearson's treatise on vaccination and Stanton's Chinese translation of it, he is said to have remarked "that the Chinese seemed much readier to resort to vaccination than the English people nearer home."[72] While this was hardly the case, Jenner was obviously pleased to learn that the descendants of his fragile cowpox virus had traveled so far and wide and with such apparent success.

As Jenner's cowpox vaccine encountered conditions and climes far from Western Europe, it took on a life of its own. In the colonies of Britain, France, and the Netherlands, the European physicians stationed there introduced vaccination and taught the technique to local physicians. But over the longer term, the capacity of vaccination to achieve the global eradication of smallpox required not only local interest and involvement, but an infrastructure that could preserve the viability of cowpox vaccine, keep track of who had been vaccinated and who had not, and distribute vaccine in an orderly and timely manner. The eradication of smallpox required not only knowledge of vaccination and access to vaccine, but sophisticated and interlocking institutions that operated and collaborated at local, national, and international levels. These institutions—which in time would indeed eradicate smallpox from the world community—would not exist for another century and a half. Meanwhile, as long as the smallpox virus existed anywhere, everyone was at risk everywhere.

In 1800, there were still many barriers that the cowpox virus could not breach. Although geography created the most obvious difficulties, the most intransigent barriers were human. Cowpox, like smallpox, was an infection. Just as the transmission of smallpox required the interaction of people and places to establish and maintain itself as a universal human disease, the transmission of vaccination required the same interaction to universally eradicate that disease. Places and people that were disconnected, for whatever reason, from the increasingly interconnected world of the nineteenth century were unable to claim the benefits of this diffusion of knowledge about Jenner's cowpox vaccine. The Japanese Islands were just such a place.

THREE

Engaging the Periphery

When Francisco Xavier de Balmis departed Canton for the long voyage back to Spain, he had extended his mission well beyond the boundaries of the Spanish empire. His ability to oversee the dissemination of cowpox vaccine had weakened as he moved from New Spain to the Spanish Philippines, to Portuguese Macao, and, finally, to the British East India Company's compound in Canton. It is doubtful that he thought at all about taking cowpox vaccine to Japan.

Few Europeans knew very much about Japan at the beginning of the nineteenth century, and Japan's knowledge about the rest of the world was also limited to a relatively small number of people. Two centuries earlier, the Tokugawa *bakufu,* the shogun's government in Edo, had made strict control of foreign information the centerpiece of its exclusionist foreign policy. Foreign trade was limited to the port of Nagasaki, chosen, in part, because of its considerable distance from Japan's political capital in Edo. Official foreign trade was limited to Chinese and Dutch ships, and the number of ships permitted to come to Japan each year was determined by the Edo government. This number decreased substantially during the eighteenth century. Japanese records suggest that the number of Chinese ships coming to Nagasaki fell from a yearly average of more than seventy to less than twenty; the average number of Dutch ships fell from five or six to one or two.[1]

Information about foreign developments usually reached Japan through the official Dutch and Chinese trading posts at Nagasaki, where Japanese officials interacted with the foreign merchants stationed there. The Dutch trading post was situated on a tiny island called Dejima in Nagasaki Bay. Dejima was connected to the city of Nagasaki by a bridge, but only a small number of authorized Japanese officials and merchants were permitted to enter the island. News from Dutch sources was translated by Nagasaki interpreters who were specially trained in the Dutch language to perform this role. On rare occasions, Japanese castaways who managed to return to Japan also brought unofficial news with them.

Under normal circumstances, information about Edward Jenner's cowpox method would have reached Nagasaki through the authorized channels of the Dutch East India Company (Verenigde Oost-Indische Compagnie [VOC]), an official arrangement established by the Tokugawa *bakufu* in the 1640s. Dutch ships sailed regularly from Holland to Batavia (today's Jakarta), and once a year ships sailed from Batavia to Japan. The pattern of trade between Batavia and Nagasaki was dictated by monsoon winds, which meant that the ships had to leave Batavia in the early summer and return in the autumn or early winter of the same year. Depending upon the weather, the trip might take one to two months.

Before ships were allowed to dock and unload, all firearms were removed, and forbidden items, such as books referring to Christianity, were censored or destroyed by Japanese officials. The items of trade were checked against the bills of lading signed in Batavia. These procedures could take up to a week or more. In addition to authorized items of the commercial trade, the Dutch ships also brought gifts for the shogun and other high-ranking Japanese officials. Requests or demands for these gifts were submitted to the Dutch a year or more in advance. Ordinary Japanese officials who handled the Dutch trade, however, were forbidden to accept gifts from any foreigner.[2]

Incoming ships also brought replacements for the Dutch merchants and took those being replaced back to Batavia. The top officials on Dejima were the Opperhoofd (Director), Scriba (Secretary), Pakuismeester (Warehouse Supervisor), and Oppermeester (Physician). The Dutch ships returned to Batavia with copper, Japan's main export commodity, plus detailed accounts of daily activities that had been recorded in the *Dagregister*, and correspondence written the previous year.

During the 1790s, the economic and political fortunes of the VOC seriously began to fail, and in 1796 the government of the Netherlands assumed the company's debts. The Dutch government revoked the VOC's charter in 1796, but sought to continue the company's special trading arrangement with Japan. To do so, the Dutch merchants had to keep the fact that the Japan trade was now in the hands of the Dutch government from the Japanese government. The Tokugawa *bakufu* was adamantly opposed to conducting any trade with foreign governments.

Despite these difficulties, the Dutch merchants were able to negotiate a new trading agreement that reduced their expenses. The important economic issues for the Dutch were longer tenures for the Dutch personnel at Dejima and the abolition of the expensive annual court journey to Edo.[3] Initially, the Japanese had required that a new Factory Director be sent to Japan each year: ". . . if the Dutch wished to trade with Japan, a new *opperhoofd* should come every year to bring the news of the world to the Shogun."[4] Frequent and regular turnover in the office of the Opperhoofd also ensured up-to-date reports on world events, and prevented the development of friendly relationships between the Dutch merchants and Japanese officials. However, in 1794, the Japanese accepted the Dutch proposal that the Opperhoofd need not be replaced every year.[5]

The Japanese also agreed to reduce the frequency of court journey to Edo, the most burdensome of the Factory's expenses. Beginning in 1794, the court journey was required only every fourth year, but requested gifts and reports had to be brought to Edo every year by two Nagasaki officials and a senior Dutch interpreter who acted on behalf of the Dutch.[6]

The longer tenures for the Dutch Factory directors meant that the Dutch Opperhoofd remained in Nagasaki much longer than before, and it meant that he would have an opportunity to become better acquainted with local officials and customs. Conversely, the curtailing of the court journey meant less frequent contact between the Dutch and the shogun's officials in Edo. The "news of the world" previously brought to Edo by the Dutch would now be filtered through Japanese officials and the Nagasaki interpreters.

While the Dutch and Japanese were negotiating these matters in Japan, events that would have international repercussions were taking place in

TABLE 3.1

Western ships entering Nagasaki, 1790–1820

Year	Place	Nationality of Ships by Year				
		Dutch	American	Russian	British	Other
1790	Nagasaki	1				
1791	Nagasaki					
1792	Nagasaki	1				
	Ezo/Kuriles			1		
1793	Nagasaki	1				
	Ezo/Kuriles			1		
1794	Nagasaki	1				
1795	Nagasaki	1			1	
1796	Nagasaki	1			1	
1797	Nagasaki		1			
1798	Nagasaki		1 (1a)			
1799	Nagasaki		1 (1a)			
1800	Nagasaki		1			(1b)
1801	Nagasaki		1			
1802	Nagasaki	1	1			
1803	Nagasaki		1			(1c)
1804	Nagasaki	2		1		
1805	Nagasaki	1				
1806	Nagasaki		1			1 Bremen
	Ezo/Kuriles			1		

Europe. Napoleon had started his march across Europe, conquering the Netherlands and incorporating Holland into the expanding French empire. These events signaled the beginning of open hostilities between the British and the Dutch: the British navy blockaded Dutch ports and began to seize Dutch ships sailing to the East Indies. Only a few Dutch ships were able to reach Batavia or Japan after 1800. The Dutch colonial government at Batavia responded by hiring neutral ships to carry the Japan trade. In the late eighteenth and early nineteenth century, neutral ships belonging to other Western nations carried the Dutch trade between Batavia and Nagasaki, and the chartered ships of these nations sailed into Nagasaki Bay flying the Dutch flag. The Dutch merchants chose not to report the defeat of Holland by Napoleon or reveal the nationalities of the ships coming to Nagasaki to the Japanese government.

Table 3.1 lists the number and the nationality of the foreign ships that entered Japan's ports between 1790 and 1820.

Table 3.1 (continued)

Year	Place	Nationality of Ships by Year				
		Dutch	American	Russian	British	Other
1807	Nagasaki		2			1 Denmark
	Ezo/Kuriles			1		
1808	Nagasaki				1	
1809	Nagasaki	1				
1810	Nagasaki					
1811	Nagasaki				1	
	Ezo/Kuriles			1		
1812	Nagasaki					
	Ezo/Kuriles			1		
1813	Nagasaki				2*	
	Ezo/Kuriles				1	
1814	Nagasaki				2*	
1815	Nagasaki					
1816	Nagasaki					
1817	Nagasaki	2				
1818	Nagasaki				1	
1819	Nagasaki	2				
1820	Nagasaki	2				

SOURCES: Shunzō Sakamaki, "Japan and the United States, 1790-1853," *Transactions of the Asiatic Society of Japan*, Vol. 18, Series 2 (Tokyo: Asiatic Society of Japan, 1939), 6-11; 174-190; Hendrik Doeff, *Herinneringen uit Japan* (*Memories of Japan*) (Haarlem, 1833).
( ) Ships that entered Nagasaki under the command of British Captain W. R. Stewart: (1a) *Eliza*; (1b) *Emperor of Japan*; (1c) *Nagasaki Maru*.
*British ships disguised as Dutch ships after the British seized Batavia. These ships were registered in Japan as American ships in Dutch employ.

These extraordinary impediments to trade between the Dutch and the Japanese at the beginning of the nineteenth century, plus the proscription against contact between the Japanese and foreigners, might lead one to assume that news of Jennerian vaccination would fail to reach Japan at this time. In fact, news of vaccination reached Japan very quickly: Japanese sources indicate that the news was brought by an American ship carrying the Dutch trade. A young Nagasaki interpreter claimed he heard about a new method of preventing smallpox from Hendrik Doeff, the warehouse master at the Dutch Factory about the time that Doeff received word of his promotion to Opperhoofd in August 1803:[7]

A ship had just come into the port of Nagasaki bringing a book which Doeff examined. He told me that they had recently succeeded in taking *byō* [lymph] from a cow and planting it in a person. This method had a better success than the *jintō* [human pox] method which uses smallpox *byō* taken from people.[8]

The interpreter, Baba Sajūrō, was only sixteen years of age at the time. It is clear that he was already familiar with variolation, and that Doeff had explained that cowpox inoculation was supposed to be a better method.

Given what is generally known about the trajectory of the global transmission of knowledge about Jenner's discovery, the timing of this communication seems appropriate. The ship that carried the Dutch trade to Japan in 1803 was the *Rebecca*, an American ship out of Boston. It had been chartered by the colonial government in Batavia to carry the trade to Japan that year. Vaccination already was well known in Boston by this time, because the Boston physician Benjamin Waterhouse, a friend of Edward Jenner, had introduced vaccination to the city with much fanfare in 1799.[9]

Moreover, the Dutch physician on the *Rebecca,* Jan Frederik Feilke, newly arrived from the Netherlands, was a likely source of news about vaccination, which was already well known in Holland. The Rotterdam physician Leonardus Davids had translated Jenner's *Inquiry* into Dutch in 1801, and he had founded a society of Dutch physicians to help advocate support for vaccination. Feilke almost certainly would have been familiar with vaccination when he arrived in Japan in 1803, and he may have been the one to tell Hendrik Doeff about it.[10]

The fact that news of vaccination reached Nagasaki as rapidly as it reached other Asian port cities, despite the English blockade of Dutch ships, means that communication between Batavia and its Japanese trading post continued to function as long as neutral ships were able to go back and forth between the Dutch East Indies and Japan. The fact that a Dutch Factory employee, Hendrik Doeff, passed this news along to a Nagasaki interpreter, Baba Sajūrō, confirms the Dutch connection as an important source of foreign information in Japan. The problem in the case of vaccination was that the news went no further until much later. In striking contrast to the reception of Jenner's cowpox method elsewhere in the world, there appears to have been no reaction whatsoever in Japan. Why not?

Despite the regular visits of the Dutch to Edo for the express purpose of providing useful information to the shogun, information that had not been requested was unlikely to get much farther than Nagasaki. In 1800, except for physicians interested in Western medicine, there were few individuals in Japan to whom an interpreter—especially a young, apprentice interpreter—might communicate information about a new medical technique. While there may have been some private discussions about vaccination locally, nothing came of it until much later when Baba Sajūrō acquired more information under very different circumstances.

The names of Hendrik Doeff and Baba Sajūrō are routinely linked in Japanese accounts about how vaccination was first introduced to Japan. Since this is a book about connections, the connection between these two young men deserves consideration. Both men were unusual, and both were products of the unusual times in which they lived. Their careers were strongly influenced by the changing international scene, by unexpected complications that made their livelihoods more difficult, and by their mutual acquaintance. Each of them had a major impact on important developments in Japan having nothing to do with vaccination, yet the link between them that is always mentioned in Japanese sources about either man is the casual transmission of information about cowpox vaccination. Since both men would help build networks promoting Japanese-Dutch collaboration in the early nineteenth century, a brief introduction to their lives and the times in which they lived is appropriate.

HENDRIK DOEFF (1777–1835)

Hendrik Doeff left Holland for the Netherlands East Indies as a young man of nineteen in 1798, just before Jenner's discovery became known in Europe. He served briefly as a junior merchant in Batavia and sailed for Japan the following year on the *Franklin,* a chartered American ship.[11] Upon its arrival at Nagasaki, the crew of the *Franklin* found the situation at the Dutch Factory in a disastrous state.[12] The Opperhoofd, Gijsbert Hemmij, had died the previous year while returning to Nagasaki from the court journey to Edo,[13] and on the island of Dejima the Factory warehouses and other buildings had been destroyed by fire.[14] The Batavian government was unaware of these calamities because the *Emperor of Japan*, the ship that had been sent out the previous year, had sunk on the return voyage. In the autumn of 1799, Doeff returned to Batavia on the *Franklin* to inform the government of the grave situation in Japan. News of vaccination had not yet reached the East Indies when he returned to Japan the following spring with a new Opperhoofd, William Wardenaar. The continuing hostilities between Holland and Britain meant that Doeff did not leave Japan again for seventeen years, so he would have had no personal experience of vaccination until after he left Japan in 1817.

Accounts of Hendrik Doeff's years in Japan can be found in his correspondence, in the annual *Dagregister* reports he sent to Batavia, and in the personal memoir, noted above, that he published after returning to Holland. Doeff was an insightful observer whose colorful commentary on life in Japan provides an introduction to some of the Japanese officials who became his friends and associates. After becoming Opperhoofd in 1803, he traveled on the court journeys to Edo three times—in 1806, 1810, and 1814.[15] Doeff's lengthy tenure as Opperhoofd, longer than any other Japan Factory employee, meant that he had ample opportunity to interact with Japanese officials and scholars in both Nagasaki and Edo.

A large contingent of local Japanese officials and specially designated Nagasaki interpreters accompanied the Dutch when they went to Edo. Bearers carried the luggage, which included the many gifts to be presented to the emperor in Kyoto and the shogun and other government officials in Edo. Palanquins carried the most important officials, including, among the Dutch, the Opperhoofd, the secretary, and the physician.[16] Special medicines were regarded by the Japanese as very fine gifts, and the physician's medicine chest occupied a prominent place in the entourage.

While in Edo, the Dutch were housed at the Nagasakiya, an official residence provided for their accommodation. After the obligatory audience with the shogun, where the Dutch answered questions that were then translated by an interpreter, they were visited at the Nagasakiya by prominent *rangaku* scholars—Japanese officials and scientists, many of whom were physicians, who were interested in various aspects of Western knowledge. Doeff had learned to speak Japanese and the *rangaku* scholars had studied Dutch, but communication relied also upon the Nagasaki interpreters.

Doeff wrote about these sessions in his memoirs. He specifically mentions Baba Sajūrō, who clearly served as a link to Edo scholars interested in Western medicine and science:

> The physicians and astronomers would usually visit us three times. They ask many questions and show great curiosity. They want to know everything there is to know about medicine and medicinal herbs, and their questions to

our doctor are usually prepared in advance. The astronomers address their questions to the Opperhoofd. Their only guides are books such as Lalande's *Astronomie*. In 1810 I became friends with the first astronomer Takahashi Sampei [Kageyasu]. Usually these gentlemen would come around two in the afternoon and stay until the evening.

On my second court journey to Edo in 1810, I met a Dutch interpreter who before 1808 had been my student at Nagasaki. His name was Baba Sajūrō, but we called him Abraham. Some of his friends in Edo also wished to have a Dutch name and he asked me to do this. The first for whom he requested a name was Abraham's supervisor, the Court Astronomer, Takahashi Sampei. Because of this, I got to know Takahashi Sampei, who would visit me daily in secret.

In 1814 our friendship became even closer, and when I left Japan in 1817 he [Takahashi] gave me clear signs of his affection . . . , I gave him the name of Johannes Globius, and I gave the name Johannes Botanicus to Katsura-gawa Hōan, the first physician of the Emperor [Shogun].[17]

The bestowing of Dutch names on Japanese officials was obviously intended as a gesture of good will that seems to have been enjoyed by the Dutch and appreciated by the Japanese.[18] This practice was also useful because it helped the Dutch merchants who came to Japan later to identify friendly Edo officials. Doeff's remarks suggest that he made a conscious effort to develop good relationships, even friendships, with some of the highest-ranking members of Edo's *rangaku* establishment. Medicine was a common topic, and the Factory physician was an important participant at these meetings. Conversations between the Dutch and the Japanese physicians provided a forum in which the topic of vaccination might have been introduced. The Dutch physician A. L. Keller had discussed variolation with Ōtsuki Gentaku during a visit to Edo in the 1790s; however, except for Doeff's conversation with Baba Sajūrō in 1803, there is no evidence that Doeff spoke to anyone else about vaccination.

Doeff's major contribution to the exchange of knowledge during his time in Japan was the Dutch-Japanese dictionary he compiled with the assistance of the most knowledgeable Nagasaki interpreters.[19] The dictionary, known as the *Doeff haruma* or *Nagasaki haruma*, was based on the Dutch-French dictionary compiled by François Halma.[20] The Shogun Tokugawa Ienari commissioned the dictionary; work began in 1812; and when Doeff left Japan in 1817, it was almost finished. Dutch words, in alphabetical order, are followed by a short phrase or sentence in Dutch and a short phrase or sentence in Japanese. The *Doeff haruma* has entries in Dutch and Japanese for both "smallpox" (*kinderpokjes* and *hōsō*) and "inoculate" (inenten and ueru), respectively, but there are no entries for "cowpox" and "vaccination."[21] Since neither Doeff nor the interpreters who were stranded at Dejima had any personal knowledge of vaccination, this is not surprising. And since the disease of cowpox did not exist in Japan, the Japanese had no immediate use for the term.[22] Instead, it was Baba Sajūrō who took up the matter of vaccination.

BABA SAJŪRŌ (1787–1822)

Baba Sajūrō was born to a Nagasaki merchant family named Mitsukuriya, but little is known of his original family. At an early age he was identified as having a special talent for languages, and the Baba family of Nagasaki interpreters adopted him. Sajūrō had an older brother, Baba Tamehachirō, who was a junior interpreter (*ko-tsūji*) in 1800.[23] Tamehachirō adopted Sajūrō as his son and heir so the latter could enter the hereditary interpreter ranks.[24] Adoptions by older brothers were not uncommon. They created a fictive father-son relationship and, in the absence of a suitable heir, made the younger brother eligible to continue the family line and occupation.

Baba Sajūrō studied under the renowned Dutch scholar Shizuki Tadao (1760–1806), and two Nagasaki interpreters, Yoshio Kōgyū (Kōzaemon) (1724–1800) and his son Yoshio Gonnosuke (1785–1831).[25] Shizuki Tadao was a reclusive individual who had relinquished his own interpreter position when he was quite young to study and translate Dutch manuscripts. He took very few students. His primary interest being Western science, he wrote and translated books on subjects that included mathematics, astronomy, and geography. His most famous accomplishment was *Rekishō shinsho* (*New Book of Astronomy*).[26] Shizuki Tadao's ability to translate the Dutch language was largely self-taught. He obtained a copy of *Nederduitsche spraakkunst*, a Dutch grammar compiled and published almost a century earlier,[27] and he worked out Dutch grammatical principles as he translated. Shizuki Tadao wrote the earliest systematic texts on Dutch grammar and taught his students from these texts.

Baba Sajūrō seems to have been a natural linguist, and he progressed rapidly under his teacher's tutelage. He quickly absorbed Shizuki Tadao's understanding of Dutch grammar and soon surpassed his teacher. By age twenty he had written two treatises on the Dutch language: *Rango kanriji kō* (*About Dutch*

Articles) and *Rango shubi sesshi kō* (*About Dutch Prefixes and Suffixes*). He pioneered new ways to teach the Dutch language, and, unlike his teacher, he would teach a generation of Japanese physicians and scholars to read and translate Dutch. While in Nagasaki, Baba Sajūrō studied both Dutch and French with Hendrik Doeff, and the two men formed a strong mutual attachment.

Under normal circumstances Sajūrō would have remained in Nagasaki, served as an interpreter and official translator of commercial documents, and taught Dutch to the Japanese scholars who increasingly came to Nagasaki to learn how to translate Dutch writings. But in 1804, a series of stunning attacks on Japan's sovereignty led to Baba Sajūrō's professional advancement as a translator and linguist, and to new sources of information about Jennerian vaccination.

* * *

In August 1803, a Russian naval expedition left Kronstadt under the command of Captain Ivan F. Krusenstern to begin the first Russian voyage around the world. On October 20, 1804, one of the ships, the *Nadeshda*, sailed into Nagasaki Bay with Krusenstern, 88 crew members, four Japanese castaways, and Nicolai Petrovich Rezanov (1764–1807), a special envoy of the Russian government. The Japanese authorities had been alerted by the Dutch and the Russians were expected. The diplomatic formalities were handled by two Nagasaki commissioners jointly representing the Tokugawa government. The Russians presented official documents stating that Russia was seeking friendly relations with Japan, an opportunity to return several Japanese castaways, and a formal trade agreement with the Japanese government. They presented a permit to enter the port of Nagasaki that had been granted more than a decade before to a Russian explorer in Ezo (today's Hokkaido). The Russians requested permission to proceed to Edo to present their request to the shogun.[28]

The Russians may have been expected, but they were not welcomed. Communication presented a major problem: the documents presented were written in Russian, in Manchu, and in an undecipherable version of Japanese. Eventually, a Russian surgeon on the *Nadezhda* who knew a little Dutch wrote a Dutch version of the Russian requests, which the Nagasaki interpreters then tried to translate into Japanese. Needless to say, these problems presented great difficulties for the Nagasaki officials, and they sent to Edo for instructions.[29]

Four months later, the Russian ship finally was permitted to enter the port of Nagasaki. Its crew was sequestered and closely guarded in an isolated compound, and the Russians were told to wait for further orders from Edo government. Finally, on March 12, 1805, word arrived from Edo. Permission for the Russians to proceed to Edo was denied: Japan had no interest in trading with Russia, and under no circumstances were Russian ships to approach Japan again. *Bakufu* officials reiterated Japan's policy of "shell and repel," emphasizing that no foreign ships would be allowed to enter any Japanese port under the pretext of returning Japanese castaways. Castaways could be returned only through the Dutch. The gifts sent by the Russian Tsar Alexander I were rejected. The *Nadeshda* would be provided with provisions for two months and must depart immediately.

The Russians were furious. Rezanov vowed to avenge these insults to the Russian tsar, and as the *Nadezhda* proceeded northward through the Sea of Okhotsk, he observed that no Japanese troops were stationed on the northern shore of Ezo or on the island of Saghalien (Japanese: Karafuto). (See Map 3.1.) During the next two years, Rezanov devised a plan to punish the Japanese. He instructed two Russian naval officers, Nikolai Khvostov and Gavriil Davydov, to drive the Japanese off Sakhalin, destroy their installations, and take the natives of the island under Russian protection. If possible, they were to take several prominent Japanese as hostages to impress upon Japan the benefits of good relations with Russia.

The first raids on the Japanese settlements took place in Aniwa Bay in southern Karafuto on October 1806. Khvostov burned villages, plundered everything in sight, and kidnapped several Japanese guards. The following spring, claiming they had come to liberate the Kurile Islanders from the tyranny of the Japanese, the Russians did even more damage. Khvostov and Davydov raided grain and ammunition warehouses and burned Japanese settlements and government offices on the islands of Etorofu, Uruppu, and Karafuto. They killed several Japanese, took hostages, and captured four Japanese vessels, two of which belonged to the shogun. It was a complete rout: the Japanese had shown no ability to defend themselves.

Khvostov and Davidov ended their attacks on June 7, 1807, and headed back to Okhotsk. They left letters stating that the raids were a consequence of the treatment the Russians had received in Nagasaki, and that greater hostilities would follow if trading privileges were not granted. One of the hostages, a *bakufu* guard named Nakagawa Gorōji, who had been on duty when Etorofu

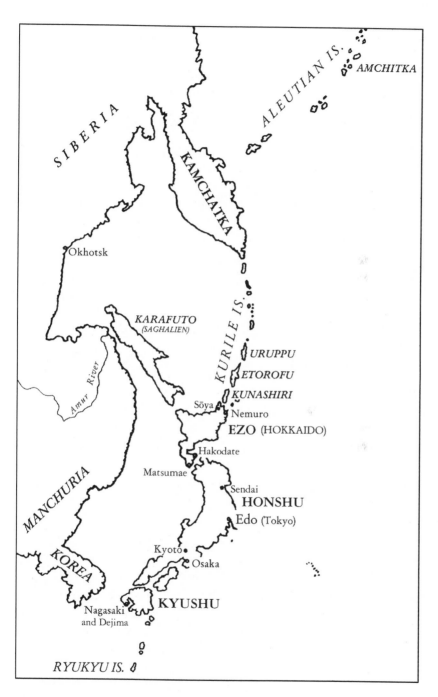

Map 3.1. The Pacific Northwest.

Island was attacked, was taken to Siberia. He would remain in Russia for the next five years.[30]

The Russian government had no knowledge of the attacks on the northern islands until they were over, and when Khvostov and Davidov returned to Okhotsk, they were arrested and imprisoned. The Russian Admiralty charged "misuse of authority by the commanders as evidenced by the seizing of tremendous riches which they have brought from Japan," and the charges led to the court martials of both men.[31] The Japanese government, however, regarded the attacks as an act of the Russian government; and, in the absence of any diplomatic relations between the two countries, the Tokugawa *bakufu* had no means of learning otherwise. Nevertheless, one thing was abundantly clear: Japan was grossly unprepared to defend itself against a hostile and well-armed neighbor on its northern frontier. The *bakufu* began to reconsider its approach to foreign policy.

The territories that encompass northern Japan and the Kurile Islands were important fishing grounds for the Ainu residents of Ezo and for the Russians and Japanese who inhabited this region of the North Pacific. Before the Russian attacks of 1806 and 1807, the inhabitants of the region had more or less decided things for themselves with little interference from the *bakufu* in Edo. They made informal trading agreements and handled the exchange and repatriation of castaways from Russian and Japanese ships lost at sea. The Edo government tended to ignore developments in the region except when serious problems demanded special attention. The *bakufu* had delegated some of its authority in Ezo by giving *daimyō* status and control over the southwestern part of the island closest to Honshu to the Matsumae clan. This arrangement gave the shogun official representation in Ezo but relieved the Edo government of involvement in local affairs.

Clearly these policies would no longer suffice. Russia's eastern expansion had reached the Sea of Okhotsk in the late eighteenth century, and Russian commercial and military expeditions were beginning to explore Karafuto and the Kurile Islands, which stretch northward from Ezo to Kamchatka. Russian ships had been approaching these islands off and on for half a century, but heretofore they had caused few problems. Contacts were handled by local officials after consultation with the *bakufu,* whose responses to unauthorized foreign intrusions had been inconsistent, but major problems had been avoided.

In the aftermath of the Russian attacks of 1806 and 1807, two new strategies were employed to deal with the problem of unwanted foreigners and foreign ships. First, the *bakufu* tightened security on the northern island by increasing surveillance of the Ezo lands beyond the Matsumae domain—territories called the Ezochi (Ezo lands)—which the Japanese had not attempted to control previously, and it sent Japanese officials to northern parts of Ezo. Among these officials was Baba Tamehachirō, Baba Sajūrō's older brother.

In 1804, when the Rezanov mission arrived in Nagasaki, Baba Tamehachirō was thirty-five years old, and he was still a Dutch interpreter-in-training. For some reason, he had been chosen to translate the Russian documents stating Rezanov's demands. How much Russian Tamehachirō could have known is unclear, but this experience seems to have brought him to the attention of his superiors. In 1805, he was promoted to junior interpreter rank (*ko-tsūji*) and summoned to Edo. That same year, Tamehachirō and the senior interpreter (*ō-tsūji*), Motoki Shōzaemon, were sent to Ezo to investigate the situation in the northern islands.[32] In 1808, Tamehachirō was appointed to a new official post at Sōya, on the northern coast of Ezo.

A second *bakufu* initiative addressed the problem of the government's profound ignorance of developments beyond Japan. Russia was not the only threat to Japan, and Ezo and the northern islands were not the only points of vulnerability. In October 1808, the *Phaeton*, a British frigate, sailed into Nagasaki harbor, seized Dutch hostages, and threatened Japanese officials. It was essential that the Japanese government learn more about the foreigners who were appearing along their shores. Although it was the function of Dutch Factory personnel at Dejima to inform the Japanese government about foreign developments, the Dutch, who were no longer receiving news from Batavia, were in a poor position to discern what the Russians and the British were up to. In 1807, no Dutch ships had come to Japan for three years.

Both of these government initiatives affected Baba Sajūrō directly. The only Japanese even remotely capable of assembling and assessing information from foreign sources were the Nagasaki interpreters and *rangaku* scholars studying various aspects of Western science and medicine. By the nineteenth century, the isolation the *bakufu* had imposed on Japan two centuries earlier had made it completely dependent upon the few Japanese who could speak or read Dutch, and even the most avid and talented scholars were severely limited in their ability to learn about the state of world affairs.

To address this weakness, in 1808 the *bakufu* established a Bureau for the Translation of Western Books (Bansho wage goyō) at the Tokugawa Astronomy

Observatory (Tenmondai) in Edo's Asakusa district.[33] The *bakufu* appointed the Edo physician, Ōtsuki Gentaku, the acknowledged founder of the *rangaku* movement, as Director of the Translation Bureau. Gentaku then chose prominent Dutch scholars, the majority of whom were physicians, to work under him. In addition to the physicians, the translation team included some astronomers, botanists, and Dutch interpreters. In essence, the Bansho wage goyō was a Tokugawa in-house research team: its task was to translate Western books on subjects considered of interest and importance to the Tokugawa government. However, given the government's ignorance about foreign matters, the *tenmonkata*,[34] as those who worked at the Tenmondai were called, were pretty much on their own to decide which books, among those available to them, should be translated into Japanese.

One consequence of the creation of Translation Bureau at the Tenmondai was that it brought Japan's *rangaku* scholars under the surveillance of the Tokugawa government for the first time. Clearly this was the *bakufu*'s intention. It was no longer appropriate to have Japan's most capable translators situated far from the seat of government in Nagasaki, interacting with Dutch merchants who now were staying for long periods and becoming much more familiar with Japan. Of even greater importance in the longer term, perhaps, the creation of a Translation Bureau in Edo institutionalized the work of the *rangaku* scholars within the *bakufu*. Setting Japanese scholars at work on joint projects allowed them to share information and to develop positions and attitudes that might be at odds with *bakufu* policy. The Tenmondai and the Translation Bureau were beginning to take up the functions of a university, and the *tenmonkata* were acting like colleagues.

In the spring of 1808, Baba Sajūrō, now twenty-one years old, was summoned to Edo to work at the Translation Bureau under Takahashi Kageyasu, the *bakufu*'s Chief Astronomer, who was translating a map of the world.[35] The choice of one so young and so junior in the interpreter hierarchy was highly unusual—so unusual, in fact, that Numata Jirō felt it necessary to consider possible reasons for this appointment. Numata Jirō believed that Baba Sajūrō's formidable linguistic ability was the first and most compelling reason. Takahashi Kageyasu needed the most capable of the Dutch translators to supervise the world map project. But there were other considerations as well, and they provide some insight into the ways that individual scholars were starting to move within existing government and *rangaku* hierarchies to form new information networks.

The second reason was that a personal recommendation certainly carried great weight. Ōtsuki Genkan, the son of the Director of the Translation Bureau, Ōtsuki Gentaku, had become acquainted with Baba Sajūrō when both young men were Shizuki Tadao's students in Nagasaki. Genkan had gone to Nagasaki to study in 1803. He had recognized Sajūrō's superior linguistic talents, and Numata believed that Genkan may have influenced his father's choice. Third, there were few good choices available. The most likely candidate for the position would have been Ōtsuki Gentaku's star pupil, Yamamura Saisuke, who was especially knowledgeable about geography. But Saisuke had died unexpectedly in 1807, leaving no obvious candidate for the position.[36]

Finally, the conventions of hereditary office may have played a role in the decision: Baba Tamehachirō's posting to northeastern Ezo opened a spot for his adopted brother, Baba Sajūrō, to take his place in Edo.[37] Whatever the reason for Sajūrō's appointment to the Tenmondai, it was considered temporary and was never made permanent. Sajūrō would spend the rest of his short life in Edo working as a translator for the Tokugawa *bakufu*.

When Hendrik Doeff learned that his able young pupil had been summoned to Edo to take a prestigious position in the shogun's employ, he was sufficiently pleased to mention the matter in his annual report to Batavia:

> The student Sazuro, son of the junior interpreter Tamifatiero, came to inform me that his father had left [Edo] one month ago for Soya, which is situated on Jeso [Ezo], and that an order from the court has arrived saying that he, Sazuro, is to go to Jedo [Edo]. I congratulated him on receiving this summons as it will contribute much to his progress. This he deserves for not only is he a very attentive youngster but also very capable in matters concerning the Dutch language. Yes, so capable in fact, that if he should ever become a senior interpreter, he surely would be the cleverest interpreter there has been for fifty years.
>
> Friday, 15 April 1808[38]

Baba Sajūrō's posting to Edo created an important intellectual and social link between Nagasaki and Edo. As part of his official duties at the Tenmondai, Sajūrō translated Western books on a wide range of topics that included geography, physics, chemistry, astronomy, medicine, linguistics, and travel literature. His translations dealt with technical topics and practical information thought to be useful to the *bakufu*, such as calendar computations, clocks,

weights and measures, the barometer, and glass manufacture. And Sajūrō became the candidate of choice for special government assignments that required knowledge of foreign languages.

Privately, Sajūrō taught some of Japan's best known *rangaku* scholars to
read Dutch at Sanshindō, the school where he tested and revised his linguistic theories. He continued to develop new approaches to foreign language
learning, emphasizing the understanding of grammatical construction as the
key. He also continued his study of Western languages other than Dutch.
Before leaving Nagasaki, he had studied French with Doeff and English
with the warehouse master, Jan Cock Blomhoff. After moving to Edo he
took up the study of Russian. His teacher was Daikokuya Kōdayū, a former
Japanese castaway who had been allowed to return to Japan. Kōdayū was no
ordinary castaway. He was a wealthy ship captain from Ise who had been cast
adrift in a storm off Honshu in January 1783, shipwrecked with his crew on
Amchitka Island in the Aleutians for four years, picked up by a Russian ship,
and taken to St. Petersburg, where he was introduced to the Tsarina, Cathe-
rine the Great.[39] He had been returned to Nemuro in northeastern Ezo in
1797 by the Finnish naturalist and explorer Adam Laxman.

The *bakufu* looked upon Japanese castaways who had lived abroad with
deep suspicion, and Daikokuya Kōdayū was interrogated at length for many
months after his return. He escaped the harsh punishment usually meted out
to returned castaways because of his knowledge of Russia, which was useful
to the *bakufu,* but he was not permitted to return to his home domain. Kōdayū's situation provides some idea of the lengths to which the *bakufu* went
to control information from foreign sources. Because of his position as an
official translator, Baba Sajūrō could take advantage of Kōdayū's presence in
Edo and engage him as a Russian language teacher. Hence, when a new crisis
involving Russia erupted in 1811, Sajūrō was one of the few individuals in
the *bakufu*'s employ who knew some Russian.

On July 11, 1811, in retaliation for the Russian raids of 1806 and 1807,
the Japanese seized a high-ranking Russian naval captain named Vasilii
Mikhailovich Golovnin, who was conducting a special exploratory mission for
Tsar Alexander I. Captain Golovnin had been commissioned to chart the Sea of
Okhotsk, one of the few remaining uncharted seas at the beginning of the
nineteenth century, and to survey and explore the Kurile Islands. Golovnin
knew about the raids of Davidov and Khvostov, but apparently he did not
know the extent of the devastation and outrage they had caused. When he and

several of his crew members on the *Diana* went ashore on Kunashiri Island, they were seized, bound, marched across Ezo, and held prisoner in the Japanese stronghold at Matsumae.

At the end of 1812, Golovnin and his fellow prisoners still had not been released, and Captain Ricord, who had assumed command of the *Diana* after Golovnin's capture, collected Japanese castaways and hostages in Russia to offer in exchange for the prisoners. Among those the Russians offered in exchange was Nakagawa Gorōji, the *bakufu* guard who had been taken hostage in 1807. While in Siberia, Gorōji had worked for a Russian physician in Irkutsk and had been taught to perform cowpox vaccination. In December 1812, when he was returned to Japan, Gorōji brought with him a Russian vaccination tract that had been published in Moscow in 1805.

This Russian vaccination tract was an official government publication.[40] It claimed that inoculation with cowpox vaccine would prevent smallpox and encouraged those who read it to take up the practice. The purpose of the tract was to educate Russian physicians about the benefits of vaccination, to explain why vaccination was less dangerous than variolation, and to instruct physicians how to perform vaccination. The tsarist government had distributed this publication to physicians in Siberia, because smallpox mortality was unusually high among the formerly isolated inhabitants there.

Nakagawa Gorōji was interrogated by *bakufu* officials in both Ezo and Edo about his observations and activities while he was in Russia, and the Ezo interrogators asked why he had the Russian publication in his possession. But they showed little interest in the contents of the book, which none of them could read. They confiscated the Russian vaccination tract, which remained in Ezo.[41]

Soon after the return of Nakagawa Gorōji, preparations began in Edo to negotiate the release of the Russian prisoners. In early 1813, the *bakufu* organized a delegation headed by a newly appointed Japanese official (*bugyō*) to handle the negotiations in Matsumae, and chose two Tenmondai scholars— the mathematician Adachi San'ai[42] and the interpreter-translator Baba Sajūrō —as members of the delegation. San'ai and Sajūrō were to learn as much as possible about Russia and Russian intentions while the Japanese still had the captives at their disposal. Sajūrō may have seen this as a golden opportunity to improve his Russian language skills.

The Edo delegation arrived in Matsumae in mid-March 1813, and within a few days Baba Sajūrō and Adachi San'ai visited the Russian prisoners. Golovnin kept a journal of his captivity which he later published, and his accounts of his interactions with his Japanese captors reveal a great deal about what the Japanese wanted to know. He wrote frequently about his sessions with San'ai and Sajūrō:

> About this time, two learned Japanese, viz. the academician and the interpreter of the Dutch language, paid us their first visit. We merely exchanged compliments, and they made no allusion to the object of their journey. They brought us some sweetmeats, and requested that we give them a French dictionary and one or two other French books.[43]

Golovnin, who was ordered to teach Russian to San'ai and the interpreters, expressed extreme annoyance at being asked to play language teacher after almost two years of captivity. But he warmed to his task as he became better acquainted with San'ai and Sajūrō:

> We were now daily visited by the Dutch interpreter and the learned man, whom we have styled the academician, because he was a member of a learned society somewhat resembling our European academies. The interpreter began to fill up and improve the Russian vocabularies: he used to refer to a French and Dutch Lexicon, for the purpose of acquiring through the French such Russian words as he did not know; he then searched for these words in a Russian Lexicon which he had in his possession. He was about twenty-seven years of age; and as he possessed an excellent memory, and considerable knowledge of grammar, he made rapid progress in the Russian language. This induced me to attempt to compile a Russian grammar for him, as well as I could, from mere recollection.[44]

Golovnin also translated French and Dutch dialogues into Russian exercises and wrote a manuscript for Baba Sajūrō to translate.

Negotiations in Matsumae over the release of the prisoners continued for another six months, during which time there were many documents to be translated. San'ai and Sajūrō were in constant attendance during these negotiations. The Governor of Matsumae requested their presence at all the proceedings so that no one could make a false representation of what had occurred to the *bakufu*. The *Diana* returned and anchored offshore Matsumae in June 1813, but in September the prisoners were moved to Hakodate. According to Golovnin, from that time Sajūrō and San'ai spent all of their time with the prisoners, even asking that their meals be sent to the house where the Russians were being held. As the negotiations began to wind down and the release of the prisoners seemed imminent, San'ai and Sajūrō worked furiously to learn as much as possible from the Russians.

> They spared no pains to obtain all the information before the *Diana* should arrive [in Hakodate]. The Dutch interpreter [Sajūrō] transcribed several sheets of Tatisschtschew's French and Russian dictionary, and he adopted the plan of translating the Russian significations of the French words into the Japanese. He thus made himself familiar with the peculiar meaning of each word better than he could have by any other method.[45]

At some point Baba Sajūrō was shown the Russian vaccination tract that Nakagawa Gorōji had brought back from Siberia, and he asked to borrow the book so that he could make a copy of it. He then asked Golovnin to help him translate it. Sajūrō would later recall these events:

> Murakami Teisuke brought a book to the Russian residence which Gorōji, a resident of Matsumae, had obtained in Okhotsk.[46] The book was about how to plant lymph [*byō*]. I remember clapping my hands and thinking: I heard about this [method] in Nagasaki several years ago, and now I am hearing about it again in this distant land of Matsumae. Not only that, I am also able to see the book in the original Russian language.
>
> I was delighted and asked Murakami for permission to take this book to my inn. Every day I took this book to the Russian residence and asked him [Golovnin] about its content. At the time, I had had only three or four months to learn Russian, so it was not easy to understand what he was saying. This took a great effort. After many days I grasped the general sense of the book.[47]

Golovnin too wrote about working with Baba Sajūrō on the translation of the Russian vaccination tract, and about Sajūrō's efforts to understand it:

> The Dutch interpreter also undertook to translate into Japanese a small Russian book on the subject of vaccination. The volume was brought to Japan by Leonsaimo [Gorōji], who had received it from a Russian physician. . . .[48]

Golovnin added in a footnote: "This translation was completed before our departure."[49]

The final negotiations were underway by autumn. Captain Ricord brought the *Diana* to Hakodate and presented a letter of friendship from the Governor of Irkutsk to the Governor of Matsumae. It stated that the raids by Khvostov and Davydov had not been sanctioned by the Russian government and that the perpetrators had been punished. Golovnin and his fellow prisoners were released to Captain Ricord on October 19, 1813, and they departed on the *Diana*.[50] Perhaps the most remarkable aspect of this brief but intense acquaintance between Vasilii Mikhailovich Golovnin and Baba Sajūrō is that each of them wrote in such positive terms about their collaboration.

Sajūrō and the other members of the Japan delegation returned to Edo and resumed their respective duties at the Tenmondai. Golovnin may have thought the translation of the Russian vaccination tract was finished, but Baba Sajūrō thought otherwise:[51]

> When I returned to the capital in the winter, I immediately took up working on the translation myself. As I think back on it now, I could not understand about a third of it. If I forced myself to translate it there would be many mistakes. If I became more familiar with the language and then worked on the translation there would be less mistakes. So I put it aside for six years. . . .[52]

Whether there was any discussion of the Russian text during those six years is anyone's guess. If Sajūrō spoke to his colleagues at the Tenmondai or in Nagasaki about what he had learned about vaccination from the Russian text, he does not mention it in his preface to the translation. Had he discussed it with others, it is not likely that he would have written about it. *Rangaku* scholars knew to be careful about their personal involvement in unofficial projects. Sajūrō's access to and translation of the imported Russian book might well have been considered illegal. The absence of an acceptable way for a *bakufu* official to safely convey information to an appropriate government official is striking.

Several years later new circumstances again forced Baba Sajūrō to consider the matter of vaccination. On June 17, 1818, the English brig *Brothers* anchored just off Uraga at the entrance to Edo Bay. Captain Peter Gordon was sailing from Bengal to Okhotsk, and he had stopped to request permission to return to Japan with cargo to sell. Once again the *bakufu* sent Adachi San'ai and Baba Sajūrō to investigate. Peter Gordon published the following account of his meeting with the two Japanese officials in the *Indo-Chinese Gleaner*:

> On the fourth day of our stay in the bay, I was gratified by a visit from two interpreters, one of whom knew something of Russian. Each of them could speak a little English, but all our communication was in Dutch. [They

were} . . . able to understand English books, by the aid of a Dutch and English dictionary, which they always brought on board with them.[53]

Baba Sajūrō wrote about this same encounter with Gordon:

In the summer of Bunsei 1 [1818], when a British commercial ship arrived at Uraga, I was ordered to board the ship for a thorough inspection. At the time, the captain took out a book, a glass bottle, and a glass plate. He explained "that the glass bottle contains cowpox scabs, the glass plate is a tool for grinding them; and the book explains the vaccination method. I have no other gift so I will present these to you." But I had to decline them.[54]

Sajūrō knew it would be a serious infraction of Japanese law for him to accept a gift from any foreigner.

This third encounter with yet another foreign national who spoke to him about vaccination convinced Sajūrō that he must think more seriously about the importance of this matter. He took up his translation of the Russian vaccination tract with renewed interest:

As I thought about it afterward, I first heard about this from a Dutch person in Nagasaki. I then obtained a book from a Russian in Matsumae. Now in Uraga an English man wants to give me a book and scabs. I had heard about this vaccination three separate times. How odd. So I again took up the translation of the Russian book. No one had translated this book before this time. I was the first to do so. Therefore, there may be many misunderstandings and mistranslations. I hope that people who come after me will correct it.

Bunsei 3, [1820] Autumn
Nagasaki *yakukan,* Baba Sadayoshi[55]

Looking back, in his introspective preface, Baba Sajūrō refers to earlier thoughts about vaccination. He had thought that ". . . before long we would obtain a foreign book with information about this method. I waited for several years. But no such book had arrived when I left Nagasaki in the spring of Bunka 5 (1808). Even now [1820] I have not heard of the arrival of such a book."[56]

Baba Sajūrō called his translation of the Russian text *Tonka hiketsu,* "How to Prevent Smallpox." The Chinese characters he chose for his title are instructive and suggest that the translation may have had some clandestine aspect. *Ton* means "to escape" or "evade"; *ka* is the Chinese character for "flowers," and "heavenly flowers" is a Chinese term for "smallpox." *Hiketsu* means both "a secret" and "a key." The literal meaning of the title, then, is "The Secret (or Key) to Escaping Smallpox." "How to Prevent Smallpox," is an acceptable English translation, but *hiketsu* may also convey the special meaning of "secret." Many medical techniques were in fact kept secret by physicians who made their living by performing them.

But keeping the knowledge of how to perform vaccination secret was not Baba Sajūrō's intention. As he states very clearly in his preface, he finished his Japanese translation of the Russian vaccination tract because he had come to believe that the cowpox method could prevent smallpox, and that its use would save the lives of many thousands of Japanese children. The purpose of translating the Russian tract into Japanese was to prevent this important information from being lost.

Apparently, however, publication was not an option; at least *Tonka hiketsu* was not published at the time. It remained an unpublished manuscript for thirty years. Baba Sajūrō signed his personal name, Sadayoshi, the name by which he was known as a child in Nagasaki, and he identified himself as a Nagasaki official (*yakukan*), not as a *tenmonkata*. Is this detail significant? Was it the way he usually signed a private manuscript? The temporary nature of Sajūrō's Edo appointment made it technically correct to identify himself as a Nagasaki official, but he may also have been reluctant to acknowledge his official name and position on this unauthorized translation.

Baba Sajūrō's translation of the Russian vaccination tract was the first attempt to document in Japanese the potential benefit of Edward Jenner's cowpox method, and to provide specific instructions on how to perform the procedure. Sajūrō died suddenly two years later.[57] It is not known whether he shared his manuscript or his thoughts about vaccination with anyone else. But whether he did or did not, *Tonka hiketsu* did not disappear. It circulated in manuscript form and was copied, possibly by colleagues or students. One copy, about which more will be said below (see Chapter 6), was sold in Nagoya in the 1830s. It was edited and published twenty years later, in 1849.

In Ezo, meanwhile, Nakagawa Gorōji, the *bakufu* guard who had brought the Russian vaccination tract to Japan, was developing his own vaccination agenda. Gorōji began to perform a procedure that he claimed was cowpox vaccination. It is impossible to verify or reject this claim, but one must ask how he might have acquired cowpox vaccine. Had he brought vaccine lymph with him when he returned from Russia? Had he found a way to procure it after he was repatriated? Most Japanese researchers conclude it is unlikely that he did either.[58]

But it makes little difference. Nakagawa Gorōji promoted vaccination as a secret medical art that only he could perform. He neither had nor sought connections with medical, scholarly, or any other networks to assist him in the distribution of cowpox vaccine or the introduction of vaccination. As noted earlier, the successful diffusion of vaccination required a broad, informed, and active network committed to procuring, preserving, and sharing live vaccine virus. Gorōji was in no position to develop such a network.

Innovations require a receptive audience. In 1800, the only receptive audience in Japan for ideas coming from the West was the growing community engaged in Western studies—the Nagasaki interpreters, *rangaku* scholars in Edo, and *ranpō* physicians who increasingly were moving to Japan's major cities. This receptive audience had two major foci—Nagasaki and Edo. As we shall see, during the next thirty years information about vaccination was transmitted, almost imperceptibly, through private, quasi-clandestine Japanese networks that eventually connected these two foci. These Japanese networks relied most heavily upon information gleaned via officially sanctioned Dutch connections.

FOUR

The Dutch Connection
Batavia, Nagasaki, and Edo

The Congress of Vienna brought the Napoleonic Wars to an end in 1815, and the Dutch East Indies were restored to the Netherlands the following year. By this time the vaccination program in Java was developing very well. As described above, the Dutch colonial government at Batavia had received cowpox lymph from the French authorities on the Île de France in 1804. The vaccine was first used to immunize the children of European and Javanese elites and family household slaves; however, when the British seized Java in 1811, a British superintendent-surgeon who conducted a medical inspection tour of Java found that native vaccinators were vaccinating children in many parts of the island.[1]

The British appointed Sir Thomas Raffles as Lieutenant-Governor of the Dutch East Indies that same year, and he gave vaccination a high priority. Raffles was a scientist who was genuinely interested in the health conditions of the native population, and he immediately took measures to extend the practice of vaccination. He implemented a centralized vaccination program in Java that oversaw the immunization of children throughout the island.

Revenues and village lands, called "Jennerian sawahs," were set apart for vaccination clinics attached to each village, and vaccinators supervised by a European surgeon were appointed to each district.[2]

In 1815, the owners of private estates and the superintendents of the administrative districts were required to see that vaccinations were performed in the territories under their jurisdiction. Sample vaccination forms were distributed to district authorities, and reporting methods were standardized and centralized. Local vaccinators were to report the number of vaccinations (both successes and failures) each month to their district authority. District authorities, in turn, were required to summarize and send their reports to one of the four superintendents of vaccination.

When the British returned the Dutch East Indies to the Netherlands in 1816, Raffles's vaccination regime was securely in place. He must have been pleased with his achievement, because when he returned to England that year, Raffles made a point of visiting Edward Jenner at his home in Berkeley to report on his successes in Java. He also spoke with a Dr. Coley of Cheltenham, who published the Raffles account in the *Medico-Chirurgical Journal* for February 1817.[3]

The restored Dutch government in Batavia continued to build on the British system, regularizing both local vaccination services and central control over those services. Vaccinations were to be performed on fixed days at fixed places each week, and district supervisors were to check the number of vaccinations against the number of births in their districts to determine how well these policies were being carried out. District supervisors were required to make inspection tours of their districts every six months, and special vaccinators were assigned to districts that were too far from a supervisor's residence. In 1820, a special Inspector of Vaccination was made directly responsible to the Director of the Medical Service at Batavia, a position that was first occupied by the physician C. Blume, and then by a Dr. Bowier in 1821.[4] The Medical Service at Batavia was now in a position to export cowpox vaccine to other parts of Asia.

This early public health program was designed not only to prevent individuals from contracting smallpox, but to contain the spread of smallpox by systematically and regularly reducing the number of susceptible people in the population. The strategy was to vaccinate immediately all known contacts of those infected with smallpox when an epidemic broke out. These policies were far in advance of their time. They were far more rigorous than most home governments could manage at the time, because of citizen opposition to mandatory vaccination. Very similar containment policies, based on immunization of contacts, would gain the support of international health organizations after World War II, ultimately leading to the eradication of smallpox from the world's population in the 1970s.

Trade between Batavia and Japan resumed in 1817, and the Dutch merchants at Dejima resumed their traditional role as the window on the world for the Edo government. The Dutch connection at Nagasaki was again the main source of scientific information from the West. Although Nagasaki had played this role since the 1640s, the number of individuals who could access this information was increasing. Japanese scholars, physicians in particular, increasingly came to Kyushu to study Dutch with the Nagasaki interpreters, and to learn about Western medicine from *ranpō* physicians who practiced and taught in and around the port city. On occasion, a physician might gain access to the Dutch Factory doctor stationed at Dejima.

With the resumption of trade in 1817, Jan Cock Blomhoff (1779–1853) arrived in Nagasaki to relieve Hendrik Doeff as Opperhoofd. It was a distinct advantage to follow Doeff, who was well liked, and Blomhoff was able to build on the good relations Doeff had established with Japanese officials and scholars in both Nagasaki and Edo. Blomhoff was already well acquainted with circumstances in Japan. He had been stationed at Batavia as a member of the military in 1808 and sent to Dejima the following year. He had served as Pakhuismeester under Doeff until 1813, when he was sent to Batavia to explain to the British, then in control of Batavia, why Hendrik Doeff refused to allow the British to take control of the Dutch trade monopoly with Japan. When Blomhoff reached Batavia, he was interned and sent off to England where he was held as a prisoner of war until the end of hostilities.[5]

Blomhoff returned to Japan in June 1817, on the first Dutch ship to reach Japan after the war, accompanied by his young wife, Titia Blomhoff-Bergsma (1786–1821), and their two-year old son, Johannes. It was forbidden for foreign women to enter Japan, but Blomhoff must have thought the Japanese would let his wife and child stay once they were there. He was wrong: they both had to leave Japan in the autumn when the ship returned to Batavia.[6]

Blomhoff was the first of the Dutch to try to introduce Jennerian vaccination to Japan. He had first-hand knowledge, which Doeff had not had, about the successes of vaccination in Europe and Java. Blomhoff had spent 1815 and 1816 in Britain and the Netherlands, and he would have known that vaccination was now an accepted way to prevent smallpox. Having chosen to bring his young son with him, Blomhoff may well have thought about vaccination before coming to Japan. Like any parent familiar with smallpox in either Batavia or Japan, Blomhoff clearly would have considered having his young child vaccinated.

Whatever his reasons, Blomhoff's personal and official correspondence indicate that introducing vaccination to Japan was a personal mission of great importance to him. Perhaps, like so many others who actively participated in the dissemination of vaccination, his intention was simply to help prevent the needless suffering smallpox was causing in Japan.

Blomhoff's correspondence indicates that his first request for vaccine was sent to Batavia in the fall of 1820. A reply, dated June 18, 1821, states that "some cowpox material and some lancets, to be used for the inoculation of children, will be sent on the ships that depart for Japan this year."[7] These items, plus a book on vaccination "for his deliberation" (and a request that the book be returned to Batavia the following year), arrived in Japan later that summer.[8] The book was a Dutch translation (1802) of H. J. Goldschmidt's history of cowpox and vaccination, first published in German the previous year.[9] Blomhoff acknowledged receipt of these items in his annual report for 1821, and reported that the Factory physician, Nikolaas Tullingh, had been unsuccessful in his efforts to vaccinate Japanese children. They had used the vaccine immediately, he wrote, but the "careless curiosity of the parents or the Japanese physicians"[10] had prematurely uncovered the vaccination sites, thereby causing this attempt to fail.

Undaunted, Blomhoff asked that cowpox and lancets be sent out again the following year.[11] This request initiated a series of communications between Japan and the colonial government that provide a clear picture of the deliberate, if slow, pace at which information and goods flowed between Batavia and Nagasaki in the early nineteenth century. Blomhoff's correspondence reflects both his personal interest in introducing vaccination to Japan, and his extreme frustration over successive failures. The Batavia government records show that the colonial authorities moved his requests competently through the colonial bureaucracy. If all went well, the minimum time for a request to be granted was about eight months.

Blomhoff's request for more cowpox vaccine in 1821 left Nagasaki for Batavia on November 21, and it was approved by the Government Council in Batavia on December 24. The Council's approval initiated a series of orders and reminders to insure that this decision would be implemented when the ships sailed for Japan six months hence. The order of December 24 went to Governor-General Baron van der Capellen, directing him "to do—just like the previous year—whatever is necessary, in accordance with the Committee for Medical Supervision, with respect to the requested cowpox material and lancets. . . ."[12] The Director of Finance received a copy of this order, and he extracted relevant excerpts to be sent to Jan Cock Blomhoff in 1822.

The following spring, in preparation for the voyage to Japan, van der Capellen was reminded "in accordance with the Committee for Medical Supervision, [to do] what is necessary for the preparation and shipment to Japan of the cowpox material and lancets requested by the Opperhoofd. . . ."[13] The Inspector of Vaccination, Dr. Bowier, included a treatise on vaccination that was sent with the vaccine.[14] In late June, the captains of the *Yonge Anthony* and *Jorina* signed contracts and invoices which specified that cowpox lymph and lancets were part of their cargo:

> I, Theodorus Azon Jacomettie, Captain of the Dutch ship *Yonge Anthony*, currently at Batavia, in order to sail to Japan, where my proper unloading will be recorded, declare that I have received on board of the mentioned ship from the Resident at Batavia: . . . For the Factory: one small box with the writing 'cowpox material and lancets'.[15]

Captain van Duivenbodem of the *Jorina* signed a similar invoice for "one small box with cowpox materials and lancets," noting in his log that "at six hours we also got a cow on board."[16] There is no description of how the vaccine was packed, nor is there anything to indicate whether the presence of the cow was related to the shipment of cowpox vaccine, but Batavia had done what could be done to ensure that *V. vaccinae* would reach Japan. The *Yonge Anthony* and *Jorina* left Batavia on June 27 and arrived at Nagasaki in late July 1822.

On August 16, the Dutch Factory clerk at Dejima, D. Gozeman, certified that the two captains had delivered their loads properly,[17] and on August 17 he declared that all items on the invoices of both ships were accounted for.[18] The vaccine had been in transit for more than two months during the hottest months of the year, and it is hardly surprising that the virus was no longer viable when it reached Nagasaki. The diligence of the personnel in Batavia and Dejima could not overcome the disadvantages of time and distance.

Blomhoff seems to have been unaware that the viability of the vaccine was an issue. He held two vaccination trials with the vaccine sent in June 1822, and carefully documented the outcome of these trials in reports he sent to Batavia. His Annual Report of November 25, 1822, describes his abortive attempts to vaccinate Japanese children:

> Concerning inoculation with cowpox material: I have again received some of it, thanks to Your Excellency's favorable disposition, but so far it does not appear to have been effective. The [Factory] physician has tried it on several children but it did not take. Partly this was due to the fact that most of them had scabies or the marks thereof, because the whole nation is contaminated with it. Partly also to the fact that the Japanese do not have the patience to wait; they opened the bandages against the advice of their doctors out of imprudence or curiosity. Partly also because the children were not used to the Dutch and they would not let the physician come near them. But the main reason is that one is locked up here and no persons other than those who are stationed on the island may enter it. Especially no children, unless there is a good *onderbanjoost* [local junior official] who allows such. For these reasons this beneficial invention is difficult [to introduce] here. Furthermore, the Japanese are very indifferent, despite the terrible havoc this contamination causes among their compatriots. Of this I obtained a most vivid image during [the court] journey: almost no town from Miako [Kyoto] to Edo that I passed through was without an encounter with a crowd of people who had been subjected to the disease and who walked or were carried about with its effects—a nasty and disgusting sight.[19]
>
> This year I will try instructing the Japanese on this method to see how much progress can be made. For this reason I will request a quantity of the material next year. . . .[20]

Unlike in 1821, there had been no hurry to use the vaccine. The vaccination attempt described above was made in November 1822, just before the ships returned to Batavia. It was fortunate that the vaccine was *not* viable, because children with scabies would have been poor candidates for vaccination. They might very well have broken out with cowpox lesions all over their bodies.

Blomhoff reveals his growing frustration in this account—especially the difficulty of conducting the vaccination trials from his restricted position on the island of Dejima.

In March 1823, recognizing a need for outside assistance, Blomhoff engaged the assistance of two Japanese physicians in a second attempt to use the lymph sent in 1822. The physicians, Minato Chōan (1786–1838) and Mima Junzō (1795–1825), were ages forty-two and thirty, respectively. They were *ranpō* physicians who had come to Nagasaki from Edo to study Dutch. Blomhoff gave a detailed account of this vaccination trial in the *Dagregister*.[21]

Thursday, 6 March [1823]

Mister Minato Chōan, the physician of Awajima, Shimotsuke no Kami Sama, came from Edo to learn from the [Factory] physician and requested my permission to enter the island [Dejima].[22]

Friday, 7 March

The above mentioned doctor came and brought Mima Junzō with him. While discussing language and other trivial matters, I finally brought up the matter of cowpox. In these two persons I found much talent and intelligence. Concerning the execution of such a plan [to test vaccination] the latter in particular said that he already had a description of it and that he wants to go to Amakusa where he has heard the cows have cowpox. I made him aware of the difference between the real and the unreal kinds, and judging from what he said, I gathered that his ideas about this matter were not clear enough. I suggested that they have the book sent to me so that I can check it first, and then, at the first opportunity, test the treatment by choosing four young persons over ten years of age. . . . The Nagasaki surgeon Ikosey [Narabayashi Eisei?] agreed to supply the necessary subjects. I tried to be as clear as possible in explaining to him the benefits for humanity of the medical invention and how famous will be the first person to make it work.

The first mentioned [Minato Chōan] said that as soon as he is successful in trying it on some people, he intends to write to his Lord to ask for permission to introduce this method to the entire realm.

I refused to hand over the lymph [*stof*] even though I was asked to do so, because I want to avoid a wrong treatment that will cause prejudice and make this useful method useless. I promised them the necessary lancets and, when the ships arrive, the lymph itself as well as rewards for the test subjects who are successfully vaccinated. I hope this is reassuring.[23]

Monday, 10 March

We decided to do the vaccination experiment the day after tomorrow. They already have two subjects and I have three. In the morning Mima Junzō . . . sent me the book on vaccination by Dr. Jenner, translated by the Rotterdam physician D. [Leonardus] Davids.[24] As this work was too extensive, I gave them the work that was sent over in 1821 out of which I had extracted the main points, such as the knowledge of real and unreal pox of cows and other subjects, etc. They soon understood how it really was. The above mentioned doctor [Mima Junzō] had got the impression from the former book that horses are needed to infect the cows first, but fortunately I managed to correct this in time.[25]

The Japanese physicians were remarkably well informed about Jenner's cowpox method. They had in their possession a copy of Leonardus David's 1802 Dutch translation of Jenner's *Inquiry*, which must have been brought to Japan previously. How they came to have a copy of this book is a mystery, but they understood Jenner's ideas quite well. Jenner did indeed believe that horse-pox, or "grease" was the source of the infection in cattle, a theory Jenner developed in depth in his *Inquiry*: "That the disease produced upon the cows by the colt and from thence conveyed to those who milked them was the *true* and not the *spurious* Cow-pox, there can be scarcely any room for suspicion. . . ."[26] Rather, it was Blomhoff who was unfamiliar with Jenner's *Inquiry* and thought that they were misinformed.[27]

Not only had Minato Chōan and Mima Junzō read and understood what Jenner had written, but they appear thoroughly convinced that Jenner's technique would work. They were eager to try vaccination and were looking for cattle infected with cowpox in Japan. Moreover, they intended to recommend the procedure to their domain lords, whom they must have thought would be receptive. Given their understanding of the importance of vaccination, they must have been delighted to have an opportunity to assist the Dutch doctor. Unfortunately, the only vaccine available was the vaccine sent in June 1822, which had already failed.

Blomhoff's account continues:

> Wednesday, 12 March
>
> The above mentioned physicians came and in their presence and mine the doctor N. Tullingh vaccinated three persons. The first was the Clerk Cornelis Valentijn van Bemmel, twenty-two years old, born in Amsterdam; the second was a girl {name not legible}, ? years old, born in Nagasaki; the third was a boy brought by Junzō, named Suzoo, seventeen years old, born in Amakusa. The first got three punctures in each arm, one being washed with lukewarm water; the second got punctures in the left arm, and the third got three punctures in each arm like the first.
>
> I then entertained the doctors and gave each of those vaccinated a present in the presence of the island's first and second *ottonas* {ward officials on Dejima}, the Junior Interpreter, Saksfsaburo [Nakayama Sakusaburō], and the doctor Coseij [Yoshio Kōsai?]. Everything that happens will be written down.[28]

Blomhoff was making a serious effort to conduct this trial like a scientific experiment; however, the "children" who were volunteered for the experiment were hardly ideal subjects. The number of volunteers was smaller than anticipated, and most young men of seventeen and twenty-two would already have had smallpox. Even so, it was an opportunity for Blomhoff to demonstrate how vaccination was performed and to engage the interest of the Japanese physicians, who possibly might help him when fresh vaccine arrived from Batavia. And he knew it was important to document the procedure carefully: to record the names and ages of the participants, to have official Japanese witnesses on hand, and to offer a reward for participation. But it was all to no avail:

Tuesday, 18 March

The doctors came again and said the inoculations did not work.[29]

Thursday, 20 March

Most of the puncture marks have disappeared.[30]

Although Blomhoff's accounts of the vaccination experiments in March 1823 give the impression that he was acting in earnest to test the vaccine under better circumstances, his intent may simply have been "instructing the Japanese on this method," as he had promised to do in his earlier report to Batavia.

Jan Cock Blomhoff expected the next shipment of cowpox vaccine to arrive in 1823; however, he was about to be replaced and would have no further opportunity to introduce vaccination to Japan. In Batavia, a government memo dated May 12 suggests that the business of sending cowpox lymph to Japan had now become routine: the Head of the Medical Service was ordered "to prepare a quantity of cowpox material for Japan—*such as is done annually*—and to give this to Dr. Siebold who is about to go there, so that it may be transported there in accordance with the request of the Opperhoofd of Japan [Blomhoff]."[31] The memo included a reminder to Blomhoff to return the Dutch translation of Goldschmidt's book on the history of cowpox which had been sent to him in 1821.

Jan Cock Blomhoff's tour of duty in Japan ended in the fall of 1823. He had succeeded in bringing the Netherlands trade with Japan to its pre-war levels,[32] and he had consolidated the personal relationships with the Japanese officials and scholars initiated by his predecessor.[33] He was clearly very popular: gifts and numerous letters, written in Dutch, were sent to Blomhoff by his Japanese acquaintances during his tenure as Opperhoofd and even after his departure. These letters can be found in the archives of the Japan Factory at The Hague.[34]

This archive contains 111 letters written in Dutch to Jan Cock Blomhoff by his Japanese acquaintances between 1822 and 1826. Among them is a farewell letter from Mima Junzō, asking Blomhoff to send more vaccine, and promising to publish a treatise in Blomhoff's name if vaccination succeeded.[35]

Blomhoff's vaccination experiments may have failed, but Junzō's enthusiasm, expressed in this letter, guaranteed that news of his experiments would circulate among associates of the two doctors who had assisted him. Both Minato Chōan and Mima Junzō had close connections with *ranpō* physicians and *rangaku* scholars in both Nagasaki and Edo.

The arrival in 1823 of the new Opperhoofd, Johan Willem de Sturler, and the German physician, Philipp Franz von Siebold (1796–1866), signaled a major shift in the policies of the Netherlands government toward its relationship with Japan. Von Siebold's background was unlike most of the Factory physicians who had preceded him. With a few exceptions, most of the Dutch Factory doctors had been trained at the Dutch military college in Utrecht. Von Siebold had been specially chosen by the Dutch king, but he came from a prestigious, academic medical family, and he was unusually young. He had only recently completed his medical education at the University of Würzburg, where he studied natural history, botany, and zoology, and where he trained as a medical clinician and surgeon.[36] With the help of his family connections, at age twenty-six, von Siebold secured a position at The Hague as court physician to William I of Holland. He soon received a commission as Surgeon Major in the Dutch Army Medical Corps.[37]

William I of Holland, known as the Merchant King, planned to reorganize the Dutch trade in the Pacific, including the trade with Japan. When the British left in 1816, he had sent Baron van der Capellen, who also saw the Dutch trade monopoly with Japan as an asset, to Batavia as Governor-General. Van der Capellen hoped to better the terms of trade by learning more about Japan's resources, people, politics, and customs. He also wanted to spread "clearer concepts of European culture, art, and science to Japan."[38] Philipp Franz von Siebold was viewed as the perfect candidate to carry out these tasks. His family background, his qualifications as a physician, and his education in the natural sciences and humanities meant that he was well qualified to carry out the Dutch government's new agenda in Japan.

University-trained physicians were rarely interested in an obscure post like Dejima: the normal tour of duty in Japan was now four years, and there was very little to do. However, the opportunity to go to Japan had enormous

appeal for von Siebold. He was strongly influenced by the scientific work of
Alexander von Humboldt, whose reports of his explorations and scientific research in South America began to be published in Europe in 1807. Von Siebold was also familiar with the major scientific explorations Joseph Banks and
others had organized to assess the resources of the Pacific. He wanted to
undertake similar research in Japan, about which little was known, and to introduce this new knowledge to Europe. Von Siebold had no way to know that
his personal agenda intersected nicely with the intentions of Japan's *ranpō*
physicians and *rangaku* scholars who were eager to gain access to Western
medical knowledge.

Von Siebold left Rotterdam on September 23, 1822, and arrived in the
Dutch East Indies in April 1823. During his brief stay in Batavia, he read the
published works of various other explorers, including those of Kaempher, La
Pérouse, Krusenstern, and Golovnin. In preparation for his research in Japan,
von Siebold assembled books and articles on natural history, botany, and
medicine; maps; accounts of voyages and scientific explorations;[39] and medical instruments and pharmaceutical supplies with which to demonstrate
Western medical and surgical techniques. And it was he who took to Nagasaki the cowpox lymph and lancets requested by Jan Cock Blomhoff the previous year.

Opperhoofd de Sturler and von Siebold left Batavia on June 28 and arrived
in Nagasaki on August 11, 1828. Von Siebold immediately took up his responsibilities as the Factory physician, inoculating several Japanese children
soon after his arrival with the vaccine he had brought from Batavia. He wrote
to his uncle to report that he was the first to introduce vaccination to Japan,
but, in fact, von Siebold's attempt at vaccination was no more successful than
Nicholas Tullingh's had been.[40] There was a difference, however: von Siebold
knew why the vaccine had failed, and he wasted little time concerning himself
about it. Instead, he began immediately to build a network of useful contacts
in Japan—first in Nagasaki and then in Edo—to advance his government's
and his own agendas. Educating well-connected Japanese about the benefits of
vaccination would become an important strategy in his own agenda.

Von Siebold was extraordinarily resourceful. He quickly overcame the resi-
dency restrictions that Blomhoff had deplored—the way that "one is locked
up here" on the island of Dejima. Actually, Factory doctors seem to have been
able to leave the island more easily than other members of the Factory personnel, including the Opperhoofd. Dr. Tullingh had been allowed to make sick

calls to patients in Nagasaki.[41] And both Tullingh and von Siebold were granted permission to collect medicinal herbs and other specimens in nearby areas in Kyushu.[42]

Von Siebold greatly expanded these privileges. He had arrived in Japan at the high point of favorable Dutch-Japanese relations, and he had an initial advantage of being able to build on more than two decades of contacts made by Hendrik Doeff and Jan Cock Blomhoff with Japanese physicians and scholars in Nagasaki and Edo. He was not unaware of his debt to his two predecessors: "Just after I arrived in Dejima, in 1823, I came to know some excellent doctors who were staying in Nagasaki through the intercession of Cock Blomhoff. Among them was Minato Chōan, a doctor of high standing in Edo, the young Mima Junzō from Awa . . . and many doctors and scholars from all over the country."[43]

Von Siebold had another advantage that his predecessors did not have: he had personally been chosen by King William I and Governor-General van der Capellen in Batavia to carry out a program of scientific research in Japan. He had every confidence that he had the backing necessary to carry out his scientific work. Von Siebold's commission was to collect a broad range of information about Japan's resources and natural history: to survey the terrain and chart Japan's coastline; to collect, identify, document, and categorize specimens of native flora and fauna; to study the history and customs of the Japanese people; and to learn Japanese traditional modes of production. He sought to replicate and add to the discoveries of earlier explorers like Joseph Banks, James Cook, and Alexander von Humboldt. This was a tall order. Unlike those men, whose scientific projects were undertaken by teams of variously trained European experts, von Siebold had to recruit his own team in Japan. His success would depend entirely upon his ability to engage the good will and assistance of knowledgeable and cooperative Japanese scholars and officials.

Von Siebold began this formidable task by cultivating relationships with Japanese physicians in Nagasaki. His most important early contact was Narabayashi Sōken (1803–1852), a descendent of the interpreter-physician Narabayashi Chinzan (1648–1711), who had founded the Narabayashi school of Western-style medicine in the late seventeenth century.[44] The Narabayashi lineage specialized in Western surgery, and Narabayashi Sōken welcomed von Siebold as a physician with recent clinical and surgical experience who could bring Japan's physicians up to date on the latest surgical and medical techniques.[45]

Von Siebold began by taking a few Japanese students who wanted to learn about Western medicine. He was dependent on the assistance of Japanese physicians who understood Dutch, because, initially at least, he would not have known Japanese. At first he met with students at the Factory medical clinic on Dejima, but soon they gathered at the Nagasaki residence and medical school of Narabayashi Sōken and his brother, Eiken, an arrangement that required official permission. Early in 1824, von Siebold was authorized to build a small medical school and clinic on the outskirts of Nagasaki.[46] The school was called Narutaki, and students who were interested in learning about Western-style medicine came there from all over Japan.

Narutaki quickly became a center for learning about Western medicine with links to interested Japanese elsewhere.[47] Kure Shūzō lists the names of fifty-seven men who studied there.[48] Most were physicians, but botanists, artists, interpreters, and scholars with a general interest in Western science also studied at Narutaki. Many of these men were in their late twenties and early thirties, about the same age as von Siebold himself. Other similarities in their backgrounds can be noted as well. For example, von Siebold would have understood the physicians' patronage system that operated in Japan. Having served as a court physician to the king in Holland before coming to Japan, he would have understood the Japanese system in which talented physicians served as retainers to domain lords in return for office, rank, and a stipend. Moreover, von Siebold knew very well how to capitalize on the willingness of his physician-students to introduce him to their employer-patrons.

At Narutaki, von Siebold introduced the style of medical education prevalent in Europe at the time—classroom lectures on anatomy, botany, biology, physiology, and zoology, as well as clinical instruction. His best students became his teaching assistants: Mima Junzō, Jan Cock Blomhoff's assistant in the vaccination attempt of 1823, was made the school head student (*jukutō*) and he lived at the school. Other physicians helped with the treatment of patients in exchange for instruction. Rather than collecting the fees commonly charged by teachers and doctors in both Europe and Japan, von Siebold asked his students and patients to provide him with information and with specimens for the scientific collections he planned to take back to Europe.

Von Siebold's research strategy was to assign to his students "dissertations," written in Dutch, on primarily nonmedical topics.[49] Students who completed these assignments were awarded European-style "diplomas" stamped with red sealing wax. These academic procedures were unlike those found in Japanese medical schools, but they were not challenged. The student dissertations became the source materials von Siebold used to write *Nippon*, the book that would make him famous after he returned to Europe.[50]

Topics of these dissertations included Japanese midwifery, Japanese religion, and the ancient history and mythology of Japan. Mima Junzō wrote a short essay, "On the Preparation of Sea Salt." Another young *ranpō* physician from Edo, Totsuka Seikai (1799–1876), wrote essays on Chinese and Japanese methods of acupuncture and the Japanese therapy of moxabustion. Takano Chōei (1800–1850), a physician from Sendai domain, was especially prolific; he wrote articles entitled "Notes on the Tea Plant and the Cultivation of Tea in Japan," "The Ethics and Dress of Japanese Women," "The Art of Flower Arranging," "A Description of the Ryūkyū Islands," and essays on Shintō and Buddhist temples in Edo and Kyoto.[51] These student essays provided just the sort of information von Siebold had been commissioned to obtain.

Japanese flora was a subject of particular interest to von Siebold, and he designed European-style botanical gardens on Dejima and at Narutaki where he planted various herbs, plants, and trees. Kō Ryōsai (1799–1846), a Japanese botanist who was a student of von Siebold, wrote several essays on the different flora of Japan: "A Catalogue of Japanese Books on Herbs," "Descriptions and Illustrations of Ginseng Known to Japan," and "A Compendium of the Kinds of Spruce Trees Found in Japan." Ryōsai would become a prolific translator of Western medical and botanical works, and von Siebold would use what he had learned from Ryōsai in his own *Flora Japonica*, published after his return to Europe.[52]

At the end of his first year in Japan, von Siebold's research projects were developing so well that he complained to Batavia that his responsibilities as Factory physician were taking too much time away from his research. He asked that another physician be sent to Japan to relieve him of his medical duties, and that two assistants, including a draftsman, be sent to Japan to help him with his teaching and research.[53] Batavia balked at sending another physician, but a draftsman, Carl Hubert de Villeneuve, and a pharmacist, Heinrich Bürger, were sent in 1825. The former produced many drawings representing scenes in Japan, and the latter taught chemistry and physics at Narutaki; von Siebold made do by delegating some of his teaching to his most capable Japanese student-physicians.

By 1826, the year scheduled for the next court journey to Edo, von Siebold's reputation as an inspiring teacher of Western medicine had spread from Nagasaki to other parts of Japan. Von Siebold planned to meet with scholars in the cities and towns he would pass through between Nagasaki and Edo. In preparation for demonstrating medical procedures he believed would impress the shogun and his physicians, he assembled various medicines and surgical instruments, including cowpox vaccine and lancets, to take on the trip. Batavia had sent cowpox vaccine to Japan in 1824 and again 1825, but all attempts to vaccinate Japanese children had failed. Von Siebold wrote to the Inspector of Vaccine in Batavia recommending that he find a better way to transport the vaccine, but nothing came of it.[54]

The Dutch entourage left Nagasaki for Edo on February 15, 1826. Von Siebold managed to include several students who could translate for him and help him negotiate privately with the Japanese physicians and botanists he met along the way and in Edo. His successes began well before he reached Edo. He had ample opportunity to display his medical knowledge and to attract future students and academic collaborators. Japanese botanists in particular had anticipated von Siebold's arrival and sought him out. Botany was a subject of great interest to Japanese scholars, and some Japanese botanists were already familiar with the work of the famous Swedish botanist Carl Linnaeus (1707–1778). Carl Peter Thunberg (1743–1828), a student of Linnaeus, had served as the Factory doctor in Japan in 1775–1776, and he too had met interested Japanese scholars in Edo. Thunberg had published the first *Flora Japonica* in 1784, after his return to Sweden.[55] Von Siebold's knowledge of Linnaeus's and Thunberg's work, and his own interest in Japanese flora, opened the way for him to seek the acquaintance of Japanese botanists who had similar interests.

When the Dutch entourage stopped at Nagoya, Itō Keisuke (1803–1901), a local physician and botanist, called upon von Siebold at his lodgings. Keisuke specialized in *pen-ts'ao*, the Chinese system of plant classification based on their use and their external appearance. Discussions between the two men convinced Itō Keisuke to join von Siebold in Nagasaki, where he studied the European classification system developed by Linnaeus. He worked on identifying and classifying Japanese plants according to their Latin names, and he translated Thunberg's *Flora Japonica*, which von Siebold had brought with him, into Japanese.[56]

Von Siebold had no reason to be disappointed by his reception when he arrived in Edo on April 11. The same physicians, scholars, and *tenmonkata* who earlier had welcomed Hendrik Doeff and Jan Cock Blomhoff came to visit him at the Nagasakiya, the Edo residence that housed members of the court journey. He wrote about these visits in his diary entry for April 23:

> The court physicians stay with me all day. They reveal to me—in secret for the time being—their wish of having me stay in Jedo [Edo] for awhile, and they presented a plan of how this might be accepted by the shogun. Today I was asked to explain about smallpox and inoculation [vaccination] and I pursued this opportunity to present a plan for the introduction of this great benefit to Japan. I explained that I was prepared to bring the lymph from Batavia myself and to introduce inoculation to this place [Edo?] at the command of the Shogun.[57]

On April 24 and 25, von Siebold again had many visitors. They included court astronomers and physicians, among whom were several eye specialists. Von Siebold showed them his books and instruments related to ophthalmology, and he demonstrated the use of belladonna to dilate the pupil. On April 26 he gave his first demonstration of vaccination and felt he had made a good impression on his audience:

> Producing great enthusiasm with all the court physicians present, I operated today on a newborn's harelip, and vaccinated three children with this old *stoffe*, only to give a demonstration of how to do vaccination. Their mood concerning my extended stay is very favorable.[58]

He vaccinated two more children on April 27.

Von Siebold makes it clear that he did not expect a positive result from the vaccinations he performed. He had used old *stoffe*—presumably the vaccine which had been delivered in 1825 since no ship had come from Batavia to Nagasaki in the interim. He knew the vaccine he used was not viable, and he probably informed his audience of that fact in advance. But he could use the occasion to show how vaccination was performed and to answer questions about the procedure. His demonstration was a useful transmission of knowledge about vaccination to those officials in Edo who would be in the best position to do something about it. His promise to bring cowpox vaccine to Japan was rash, considering that the difficulty of doing so had already been well established; but von Siebold hoped that the shogun would be sufficiently impressed with his offer to allow him to stay in Edo after the Dutch mission returned to Nagasaki.

Von Siebold's accounts give the distinct impression that he collaborated in secret with *bakufu* officials to obtain special permission to stay in Edo for an extended period. If so, the collaboration failed, and von Siebold left Edo for Nagasaki with the rest of the Dutch entourage on the designated date of departure, May 18, 1826 (Bunsei 9.4.12).[59] But he had accomplished far more than he knew. He had been able to build upon his predecessors' ties with Japanese scholars in Edo, and he had initiated a series of events that would insure his own fame in Europe and Japan.

He also had precipitated a crisis that brought the wrath of the *bakufu* down upon himself and the *bakufu* officials who had assisted him. While in Edo, von Siebold made arrangements with several translators, astronomers, and medical scholars to exchange European medicines and medical information for maps of Japan and specific items of interest that he could take back to Europe. Some of these arrangements were honored, and certain prohibited items were delivered to him either during his stay in Edo or after his return to Nagasaki. In December 1829, as von Siebold was preparing to leave Japan, these items—maps, items of clothing—were discovered among his possessions, and this discovery led to his arrest. The Japanese officials who were involved in the exchanges with von Siebold were accused of treason; many were arrested and some were executed. Takahashi Kageyasu, the government's Chief Astronomer, and the most prominent among the thirty or so accused officials, died in prison before he could come to trial. The Translation Bureau at the Tenmondai was closed for a time, and a year later, von Siebold was deported.

The particulars of what is known as the Siebold Incident have been described elsewhere.[60] What is important here is to assess the consequences of von Siebold's interactions with his students and associates and determine the significance and duration of the connections he made during his stay in Japan. An examination of the activities of those with whom he associated makes it evident that his influence was extraordinary and long-lasting.

The Siebold Incident brought suspicion upon everyone associated with von Siebold. Remarkably, however, his arrest and deportation seem to have enhanced his reputation among his followers and acquaintances. His students dispersed, but they retained a certain celebrity status wherever they went. Those who had known and studied under von Siebold were regarded as having acquired special knowledge, and many of them committed themselves to disseminating what they had learned. As they moved to Edo and to other Japanese cities, they opened medical schools and clinics specializing in Western medicine, and they began to translate Western medical books on a wide range of subjects.

Von Siebold, unwittingly, had established what the Japanese call the Sie-bold-*ryū*. The term *ryū* refers to the transmission of knowledge from one gen-eration to the next through vertical lineages. The literal meaning of *ryū* is "river," in this case signifying a stream or flow of knowledge from a learned person to students or disciples. The concept is similar to "school of thought" in the West, but it is more personal, more vertical, suggesting an intellectual "line of descent" or "line of transmission" from a single individual.

A Japanese *ryū* refers both to a founder and to successive generations of fol-lowers. The multigenerational transmission of ideas, skills, and personal loyal-ties a *ryū* comprises was, and often still is, strengthened by marriage or adop-tion ties or by some combination of the two. Emphasis on the vertical transmission of knowledge and skills from master to pupil runs parallel to and intersects with Japan's centuries-old system of hereditary office and occupa-tion. This combination of social and intellectual connection promotes an adaptable version of primogeniture that passes family holdings and headships to a single individual, and allows merit to be incorporated into the mix as well. It was common practice in medical households, for example, to adopt an able student as a household successor, a practice that encouraged the development of strong bonds between teachers and students, masters and apprentices.

The Siebold-*ryū* was unusual. A Japanese *ryū* might have a Chinese founder, but *ryū* were only rarely associated with a Western founder, because, historically, there was so little contact between Westerners and Japanese.[61] Japanese scholars use Siebold *ryū* to identify von Siebold as the source of cer-tain Western medical knowledge in Japan and his "disciples" as the transmit-ters of that knowledge. No medical topic is more closely associated with von Siebold in Japan than vaccination, despite the fact that he played no direct role in introducing it, nor was he the first, the last, or the most diligent in try-ing to do so.

It was von Siebold's students who extended his influence after his depar-ture in 1829, and who built a network that advocated the importation of cowpox vaccine. His most ambitious students moved to Edo and joined the ranks of *ranpō* physicians who were forming an active community there in the 1830s. Membership in the Siebold-*ryū* was fixed, based as it was upon having been a student of von Siebold between 1823 and 1828. Although this might not seem to be enough time to establish an influential medical elite, the Siebold *ryū* expanded laterally. It became a network that transmit-ted medical knowledge through horizontal links connecting "colleagues" with common "professional" interests. This was no small accomplishment in a society in which there were neither colleges nor professions.

The transformation of the nascent Siebold-*ryū* into a multidirectional network made it possible for these new colleagues to collaborate and build networks across domain lines, a development that had the potential to challenge Japan's vertically constructed institutions controlled at the top by the Tokugawa *bakufu*. And after 1830, the activities of *ranpō* physicians increasingly were regarded with suspicion by the Edo government.

Von Siebold's teachings inspired his followers to begin translating Western medical texts devoted to various approaches to medical practice, including vaccination. Interested Japanese physicians had been translating Western medical books for half a century; and, in fact, the *rangaku* movement had launched with a famous Japanese translation of a Dutch anatomy text by Johann Adam Kulmus (1689–1745), initially published in German, in Danzig in 1725.[62] The Japanese translation, *Kaitai shinsho* (*New Treatise About Anatomy*), was a collaborative effort by Maeno Ryōtaku (1733–1803), Sugita Genpaku (1738–1818), Nakagawa Jun'an (1739–1786), and Katsuragawa Hoshū (1751–1809), physicians who belonged to the first generation of *rangaku* scholars. *Kaitai shinsho* was published with the permission of the tenth shogun, Tokugawa Ieharu, in 1775. Many later translations of Western medical texts were not published, but translating European medical texts from Dutch language editions became the most important activity of nineteenth-century *ranpō* lineages.

We can see a clear connection between translating foreign texts and the formation of medical lineages by examining the production of the multigenerational Udagawa-*ryū*. The Udagawa family was one of the more prominent medical lineages to transmit Western medical knowledge through a series of adopted successors.[63] The Udagawa-*ryū* provided employment, recognition, and status for several generations of Japanese medical scholars. Udagawa Genzui (1755–1797), the fifth-generation head, was the first member of the lineage to take up the study of Western medicine, and he joined the ranks of the early *rangaku* scholars in the 1770s.[64]

Udagawa Genzui studied Dutch with the translators of *Kaitai shinsho*, Sugita Genpaku and Katsuragawa Hōshu, and with their student, Ōtsuki Gentaku (1757–1827). He worked on the first compilation of the *Haruma wage*, the Dutch-Japanese dictionary compiled by Imamura Sanpaku and others and printed in Edo in the 1790s.[65] Genzui published the first Japanese textbook on Western internal medicine.[66] He died suddenly at age forty-two without having chosen an heir, and left the Udagawa lineage without a successor. Genzui's associates and students met and chose Yasuoka Genshin, his gifted student, to succeed him.[67] Genshin took his teacher's surname and became Udagawa Genshin (1769–1834), the sixth head of the Udagawa lineage.

Genshin's initial writings followed those of his teacher and focused on general topics related to Western internal medicine. In 1805, he published *Ihan teikō (A General Outline of Medicine)*, which integrated information from many different Western anatomy books. In 1811, he published an illustrated anatomical atlas as a supplement to *Ihan teikō,* and had it printed with copper plates instead of the usual wood blocks. Genshin also wrote the first standard work in Japanese on Western pharmacy.

In 1811, at age forty-three, Genshin adopted a successor, the eldest son of an Edo *ranpō* physician, who took the name Udagawa Yōan (1798–1846). This was an unusual move because Yōan was only thirteen years old at the time he was adopted. It was usually considered risky to adopt an heir at such a young age, as it was too early to assess the person's potential. Given his own experience, however, Genshin must have decided that it was more risky to wait. As it happened, Udagawa Genshin lived for many more years, and he had plenty of time to train and influence the development of his adopted son.

Genshin's goal was to train his adopted son as a translator. He told Yōan never to forget that translation is demanding and important work.[68] Udagawa Yōan first studied the Chinese classics and Chinese-style medicine, fairly standard training for *ranpō* physicians in the early nineteenth century. He wrote in his autobiography that he was not permitted to study the Dutch language for several years. Genshin maintained that "the traditional academic approach in the Udagawa family is based in the main on learning classical Chinese composition. If you lacked the ability to compose a Chinese sentence, you cannot achieve medical learning either. . . . But do not forget that translation is important work and worthy for a man to sacrifice his whole life to."[69] It was essential for Japanese translators of writings in foreign languages to know how to compose a proper Chinese sentence, because, at that time, Japanese medical works were written in *kanbun*, a Japanese version of classical Chinese.

Udagawa Yōan's education in the Dutch language began at age seventeen. His father finally relented and "made proper arrangement for me to study with Baba Sajūrō,"[70] who was considered the best teacher of Dutch at that time. Yōan showed an early interest in botany and Chinese *materia medica*, and he used Western herb books and Dutch pharmacoepia as the textbooks from which to learn Dutch. He studied the Western scientific field of botany by reading the sections of Noel Chomel's *Huishoudelijk woordenboek* (Household Encyclopedia) devoted to that topic.[71] Botany would become Udagawa Yōan's major field of scientific research and writing, and it was his interest in botany that provided opportunities for him to meet Dutch visitors to Edo.[72]

Yōan learned about Japanese-Dutch relations at an early age through his father's official connections to the *bakufu*. While still a youth he accompanied his father to the Nagasakiya when the Dutch were in Edo for an audience with the shogun. He met Hendrik Doeff in 1814, Jan Cock Blomhoff in 1822, and Philipp Franz von Siebold in 1826. Von Siebold described him as a scholar of great linguistic and scientific erudition, and although Yōan never studied with von Siebold, he would become closely associated with several of the latter's students, including Totsuka Seikai and the botanist Itō Keisuke.[73]

By age nineteen, Yōan had demonstrated his ability to carry on the work of the Udagawa lineage. He was given a sinecure as physician to the *daimyō* of Tsuyama domain (Okayama Prefecture), but he rendered his service to the Tsuyama lord at the latter's residence in Edo. At age twenty-four Yōan married the daughter of Adachi Chōshun, a prominent Edo physician whose interest was Western-style obstetrics. Having established a permanent place for himself in the Udagawa lineage, Yōan spent the remainder of his life teaching, writing, and translating Dutch books. He and his adoptive father, Udagawa Genshin, collaborated in many translation projects, including the monumental translation of the Chomel encyclopedia, which was underway at the Tenmondai.

Despite his strong association with von Siebold's students, Udagawa Yōan remained unscathed in the *bakufu*'s purges of the Edo *rangaku* scholars during 1829–1830. In fact, he publicly disassociated himself from those who were implicated. When the work of the Translation Bureau was suspended briefly in March 1829, Yōan sent a letter of appeal to the shogun:

> We had been translating Chomel's encyclopedia. We have no connection with the men captured in the Siebold Incident—Takahashi Kageyasu and the interpreters. We are innocent. Besides, we are confident that our translation is of great value to our country. Please let us resume this translation at once.[74]

The Translation Bureau reopened under a new director in 1830, but things were not the same as before the purge. There were problems getting books, and meetings with the Dutch at the Nagasakiya became more and more restricted. In a letter thanking Itō Keisuke for lending him a book on botany by P. J. Kasteleijn, Yōan writes: "We do not see any Dutch people in Edo these days, so there is no chance to talk to them or to obtain Dutch books. I am in good health and studying chemistry very hard, but I am greatly annoyed by the lack of chemistry books."[75] Despite these annoyances, Yōan continued to translate Western books and to write Japanese treatises on botany, chemistry, and medicine. His was anxious to integrate his knowledge of Chinese herbal medicine with the ideas he had encountered in Western books, and to extend his understanding of Western scientific ideas beyond those of his father and grandfather.

The scholarship of the Udagawa-*ryū* demonstrates how lineages created intellectual and generational links in a chain of transmission by building upon knowledge accumulated by previous generations. Yōan was an intellectual, not a biological, link in this chain of transmission. Having been carefully chosen and trained to continue to add to the legacy of the Udagawa, he fulfilled his mission perfectly. And he assured the continuation of the lineage by adopting Iinuma Kōsai as his successor. As Udagawa Kōsai, the latter would head the lineage's eighth generation and take the family position as a translator at the Tenmondai.[76]

The Udagawa spanned the entire Tokugawa period, bridging the transition from Chinese-style to Western-style medicine in the mid-eighteenth century. Its members participated in the shift from the exclusive study of Western surgery to greater attention to the Western medical fields of botany, chemistry, and pharmacy. Table 4.1 gives a partial list of the writings and translations produced by the Udagawa lineage over three generations, documenting the broadening range of medical and scientific subjects in which they engaged.

Miyashita Saburō credits Udagawa Genshin with translations from twenty-four European medical works and Yōan with seventeen.[77] Rarely translations of an entire work, they were translations of chapters or sections of books they were using for their own writings on medical topics. Few were verbatim translations. They incorporated an author's opinions and conclusions with their own experiments, or included gleanings from one or several Dutch medical books.[78] Many so-called translations were actually research papers that inte-

TABLE 4.1

Selected translations and books published by the Udagawa lineage

Publication Year	Translators	Author, Titles, Publication Place, and Year	Japanese Title (Subject)
1793–1810	Udagawa Genzui	Johannes Gorter, *Gezuiverde geneeskonst...*, Amsterdam, 1744	*Seisetsu naika senyō* (Internal medicine)
1805	Udagawa Genshin	Steph. Blankaart, *De nieuw hervormde anatomie*, Amsterdam, 1678	*Ihan teikō shakugi* (Anatomy)
1937 (Tr. 1811–1845)	Baba Sajūrō, Udagawa Genshin, and Yōan	Noel Chomel, *Huishoudelijk woordenboek*, 2nd ed. Leiden, 1768–1777 (Dutch tr.)	*Kōsei shinpen* (Household encyclopedia)
1820	Udagawa Genshin	P. van Hamel *Pharmacopoea hodierna...*, Utrecht, 1749	*Oranda yakkyō* (Pharmacy)
1822–1825	Udagawa Genshin and Yōan	P. van Hamel, *De nieuwe Nederduitsche apotheek...*, Leiden, 1766	*Ensei ihō meibutsukō* (Pharmacy)
1822	Udagawa Genshin	Johannes Gorter, *Gezuiverde geneeskonst...*, 4th ed., Amsterdam, 1773	*Zōho–chōtei naika senyō*, rev. ed. (Internal medicine)
1858 (Tr. 1822)	Udagawa Yōan	Az. Bowier "Beschreibung der cholera morbus," *Bataviasche courant*, 1821, n. 12	*Cholea morbus setsu* (Cholera)
1822	Udagawa Yōan	Egbert Buys, *Nieuwen volkomen woordenboek van konsten en weetenschappen*, Amsterdam, 1769–1778	*Botanika-kyō* (Botany)
1833	Udagawa Yōan	Job Baster* *Natuurkundige uitspanningen...*, Utrecht, 1817	*Shokugaku keigen* (Botany)
1837–1838/1846	Udagawa Yōan	William Henry *Chemie voor de beginnende lidfhebbers*, 1803 (Dutch tr.)	*Seimi kaisō* (Chemistry)
1860	Udagawa Kōsai	*Schatkamer voor alle standen*, Amsterdam, 1842–1856	*Banpō shinsho* (Encyclopedia)

SOURCES: Saburō Miyashita, "A Bibliography of the Dutch Medical Books Translated into Japanese," *Archives Internationales d'Histoire des Sciences* 25, no. 96 (1975): 8–72; Tatsumasa Dōke, "Yōan Udagawa: A Pioneer Scientist of Early 19th Century Feudalistic Japan," *Japanese Studies in the History of Science*, 12 (1973): 99–120.

*This Dutch book on botany, by Job Baster, was a present from Philipp Franz von Siebold to Udagawa Yōan, Miyashita, 25.

grated what had been learned from Western texts with familiar and accepted medical knowledge. As Miyashita's annotated bibliography of Japanese translations of Western medical writings makes clear, the Udagawa translations were collaborative efforts which might engage more than one member of the lineage with other scholars and students interested in a certain topic.

Yōan's later writings were intended for distribution to a larger and more general medical audience: "I decided to write my own book, *Seimi kaisō* (*Foundations of Chemistry*), in plain and accessible terms using in full the elucidative descriptions in simpler Western chemistry books."[79] The use of less erudite forms of written Japanese, as opposed to *kanbun*, became a trend in the medical writings of *ranpō* physicians. The reason for this change was to disseminate medical knowledge more quickly and broadly among physicians who wished to adopt or adapt their practice of medicine to include elements of Western practice.

While *rangaku* scholar-physicians who belonged to multigenerational lineages like the Udagawa-*ryū* were becoming interested in nonmedical knowledge about the West, physicians who had not been adopted into prestigious medical lineages were creating *ranpō* medical networks that had horizontal rather than vertical structures. These networks were based on common interests, interests that were disseminated primarily through teaching, translation, clinical experimentation, and medical practice. These newcomers to medicine would make Jennerian vaccination their *cause célèbre*.

FIVE

Constructing a Network
The Ranpō *Physicians*

Unlike Udagawa Yōan, few young men were adopted at an early age into prominent medical lineages, but there were several ways to become a physician in Japan during the early nineteenth century. Medicine provided one of the most important avenues of upward mobility for ambitious young men during the Tokugawa period; however, a successful journey along this path required astute planning, ingenuity, and appropriate patrons. *Ranpō* medicine offered more opportunities than Chinese-style, or *kanpō,* medicine, because fewer adherents were willing to undergo the rigorous training required to learn to read medical texts written in Dutch. Physicians who took up the practice of Western-style medicine often were well into their thirties or forties by the time they finished their training and began to earn a living practicing medicine. However, the long process of being educated created a broad range of contacts that opened opportunities for economic and social advancement.

The biographies of the seven *ranpō* physicians that follow illustrate the kind of personal transformations required of the men who decided to change their place in the Tokugawa social order. These men have been selected for discus-

TABLE 5.1

Ranpō physicians who participated in the vaccination network

Name	Birth/Death	Birth Status	Birth Order	Birthplace	Place of Death
Hino Teisai	1797–1859	Peasant	Unknown	Bungo	Kyoto
Itō Genboku	1800–1871	Peasant	Eldest	Hizen	Edo
Ōtsuki Shunsai	1804–1862	Samurai	Second	Rikuzen	Edo
Satō Taizen	1804–1872	Peasant	Eldest	Musashi	Edo
Ogata Kōan	1809–1863	Samurai	Third	Bitchū	Edo
Kuwata Ryūsai	1811–1868	Samurai	Younger	Echigo	Edo
Kasahara Hakuō	1809–1880	Physician	Eldest	Echizen	Edo

sion because of the important roles they played in the introduction of Jennerian vaccination to Japan; however, the strategies they employed were common to all upwardly mobile individuals during the Edo period. They made excellent use of three well-established Japanese social practices—personal referrals, adult adoptions, and marriage alliances—practices that made advancement possible within Japan's rigidly constructed class system.

All seven men were born around the turn of the nineteenth century. Map 5.1 shows the provinces where they were born, most of which were provinces far on Japan's periphery. None of the men was from a wealthy family and only one was the son of a physician. While little is known about the early years of these men, a great deal is known about their activities after age fourteen or fifteen, the age at which a young man normally left home to make his way in the world.

As Table 5.1 shows, these men began life as members of the peasant class, or as low-ranking samurai.[1] Medicine was often thought of as a career for younger sons who would not inherit the office of their fathers, but first sons might also regard medicine as a more attractive career than farming or military service at the lower end of the samurai ranks. By the end of their lives all seven had moved from their places of origin in outlying provinces to one of Japan's major cities.

Because of their prominent role in introducing Jennerian vaccination to Japan, these men were well known in their own time and are still honored today. Primary sources that document their activities have been preserved and published, and even small details about their lives can be found in local and national histories, as well as biographies. Japanese medical historians have done extensive research on these men and are still publishing their findings.

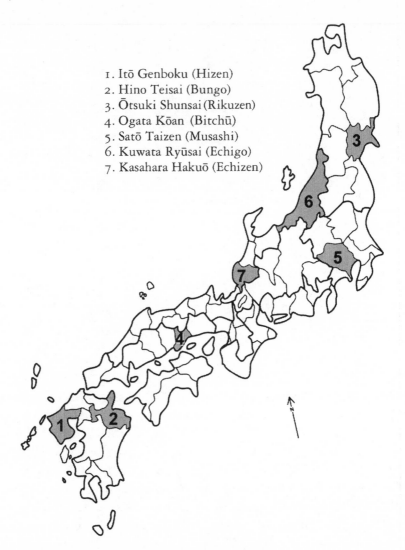

1. Itō Genboku (Hizen)
2. Hino Teisai (Bungo)
3. Ōtsuki Shunsai (Rikuzen)
4. Ogata Kōan (Bitchū)
5. Satō Taizen (Musashi)
6. Kuwata Ryūsai (Echigo)
7. Kasahara Hakuō (Echizen)

Map 5.1. Native Provinces of *Ranpō* Physicians.

Japanese biographers follow a standard format that begins by identifying an individual with the name by which he or she was best known: birth and death dates; the various names by which the person was known at different points in his life; the province, domain, district, and village where the person was born; the name, status, and occupation of the person's father and notable ancestors; important patrons; and the name of the temple where the person's memorial tablet can be found. These details create a linear account that connects an individual to his most important accomplishments: official positions, honors, and promotions; titles of books he wrote, translated, or published; and the names of well-known students and associates.

A Japanese biographical entry rarely recreates the contexts—the web of connections, associations, and relevant events within which an individual or group of individuals lived their lives. Vertical connections are given great attention, but lateral connections and intersections are often neglected. Critical interpretations are rare. The purpose of this chapter is twofold: (1) to review and assess the available and generally accepted information pertaining to the lives of seven physicians; (2) to reconstruct and integrate the contexts in which they acted, with respect to the reception and transmission of vaccination in Japan.

HINO TEISAI (1797–1859)

Hino Teisai was born in Bungo Province (today's Ōita Prefecture) in northeastern Kyushu, and little is known about his childhood. Teisai left home around age fifteen to study with Hoashi Banri, a well-known Dutch scholar. Hoashi Banri (1778–1851) was a scholar of high rank; he was born in Hiji Castle, Bungo Province, and educated in the Chinese and Japanese classics. He developed an early interest in Western science and was known for his ability to translate European scientific books written in Dutch. Hoashi Banri wrote treatises on a variety of Western scientific topics, including medicine, and he attracted talented students interested in a variety of subjects. He was known for respecting the individuality of his students and for encouraging them to follow their own interests.[2]

It is not clear whether Hino Teisai was interested in Western medicine when he began to study with Banri, but his choice of teacher suggests that he was already interested in learning about the West. As noted above, teachers who could read the Dutch language well were rare at the beginning of the nineteenth century. Dutch dictionaries had yet to be compiled, there were no Dutch grammars, and most teachers of Dutch were still learning how to read Dutch themselves.[3] This situation improved somewhat when Fujibayashi Fusan compiled and published an abridged Dutch-Japanese dictionary, *Yakken (A Key to Translation)* in 1810, prompting Hoashi Banri to acknowledge a great debt to the compiler.

In the early 1820s, after Hino Teisai had studied with Hoashi Banri for several years, he went to Nagasaki. He was in Nagasaki when Philipp Franz von Siebold arrived in August 1823 and was one of his first students at Narutaki.[4] Teisai remained in Nagasaki for several years after von Siebold's dramatic deportation at the end of 1829. In 1833, at age thirty-seven, he gained the backing of Koishi Genzui, an influential *rangaku* scholar in Kyoto, and moved to the capital where he opened a medical practice and school focusing on Western-style medicine.[5] Teisai would remain in Kyoto for the rest of his life, but during his long residence in Nagasaki he had established lasting relationships with the Dutch and Chinese interpreters and *ranpō* physicians like Narabayashi Sōken. These relationships remained a part of his personal and professional network throughout his life.

ITŌ GENBOKU (1800–1871)

Itō Genboku was also from Kyushu. He was born in Nihiyama, Hizen Province, in 1800, the eldest son of a poor tenant farmer.[6] Nihiyama was a small village in Saga domain, which was under the jurisdiction of the Nabeshima lord. Genboku began his medical career in 1815 as an apprentice to Furukawa Sa'an, a *kanpō* physician who practiced in a neighboring village. When Genboku's father died three years later, leaving his family in considerable debt, Genboku became the head of household. He set up a clinic in the family home and obviously did very well. By 1822 he had paid off his father's debts and bought the rice fields his family had been cultivating as tenant farmers.

Having fulfilled his responsibilities as the eldest son, Genboku transferred the family headship to a younger brother and left Nihiyama for the nearby castle town of Hasuike. There he studied medicine with Shimamoto Ryūshō (?–1848), a physician whose family had practiced *kanpō* medicine for four generations. Shimamoto Ryūshō's physician father had introduced him to Chinese-style medicine, but Ryūshō also went to Nagasaki to study with a Dutch interpreter. When he returned to Hasuike in 1818, he opened a private academy specializing in *ranpō* medicine, and several known scholars of Western medicine studied with him.[7] Although Genboku spent less than a year studying with Shimamoto Ryūshō but he must have made a good impression, because in 1822 he left for Nagasaki with a letter of introduction to Inomata Denjiemon, one of the senior Nagasaki interpreters.[8] He was twenty-one years old.

This chronology provides few clues about why Itō Genboku chose to study *ranpō* medicine. Had this been his plan all along? Was he influenced by some person or event before he left Nihiyama? It was not unusual for *ranpō* physicians from small villages to begin their medical training as apprentices to local *kanpō* physicians, because few small villages had *ranpō* physicians. Was Genboku influenced by Shimamoto Ryūshō, who may have been his first contact with someone who had studied *ranpō* medicine? Or was the primary purpose of Genboku's short period of study with Ryūshō to establish a connection with a teacher in Nagasaki? Whatever his motivation, Itō Genboku was an extremely determined and ambitious young man; unlike Hino Teisai, he moved rapidly through the stages required to call himself a *ranpō* physician.

Itō Genboku's introduction to Inomata Denjiemon would prove to be enormously beneficial. A proper letter of reference was essential to acquiring an excellent teacher of Dutch, but good introductions also helped one find lodging and people with common interests and goals. Genboku's letter of reference was an introduction into the society of a select group of young men who were or would become prominent *ranpō* physicians. Genboku's actions on his arrival in Nagasaki are well documented. He sought accommodation at Anzen-ji, a Buddhist temple where he did menial work in return for food and lodging. He studied Dutch and attended lectures on "Dutch" subjects at Inomata Denjiemon's school when he was off duty; and when he had proved himself, he was invited to live at the Inomata residence and work for his tuition.[9] This type of arrangement was fairly common: students frequently boarded at the homes of their teachers and lived at their place of work.

Itō Genboku had been studying in Nagasaki for about a year when von Siebold arrived in 1823. Like Hino Teisai he was one of von Siebold's first students at Narutaki, but unlike Teisai he studied with von Siebold for only a short time. It is difficult to determine what either Teisai or Genboku learned from the German physician. Von Siebold does not mention either of them in his writings, nor do they seem to have written essays for him or to have received special diplomas.

Apparently Genboku was a member of the entourage that accompanied von Siebold on the court journey to Edo in 1826. If so, his inclusion should perhaps be attributed to arrangements made by his teacher, Inomata Denjiemon.[10] Itō Sakae claims that Inomata Denjiemon arranged for Genboku to accompany his party because he thought highly of him and regarded him as a potential son-in-law. The Inomata party included Denjiemon's wife; his son, Inomata Genzaburō, also a Dutch interpreter; and his daughter, Teru. When they reached Numazu, a short distance from Edo, Denjiemon became critically ill and died after making a deathbed request that Genboku marry his daughter and look after his family. The bereaved group continued on to Edo where Genboku took up lodging at the Tenmondai in Asakusa, an arrangement that must have been made in advance by Denjiemon.[11]

The Tenmondai was an ideal place for Genboku to meet Edo *rangaku* scholars and physicians who had been working on the shogun's translation projects there for more than a decade. For a young, unknown physician from Kyushu, it was a propitious entrance into Edo society. Given Genboku's youth and status, he would not have been among the high-ranking physicians for whom von Siebold gave his demonstration of vaccination at the Nagasakiya. But Genboku did not need to witness this demonstration. He would already have known about vaccination from von Siebold's teachings and from the physicians in Nagasaki who had been involved in Blomhoff's vaccination experiments. It seems likely, however, that he would have learned about the demonstration, because it made a great impression on the Edo physicians who witnessed it.

Being identified with von Siebold and the court journey of 1826 paid enormous dividends for Genboku, whose goal was to establish himself as a *ranpō* physician in Edo. His connection to the Inomata family provided links to physician-translators at the Tenmondai, and he was able to meet the shogun's astronomers, cartographers, and foreign-language scholars working at the Translation Bureau. When von Siebold returned to Nagasaki with the Dutch embassy on May 18, Itō Genboku remained in Edo.[12] When Genboku was ready to return to Kyushu, his brother-in-law, Inomata Genzaburō, asked him to deliver a sealed document to von Siebold in Nagasaki. This document may have been Ino Tadataka's map of Ezo and Karafuto (Saghalien), which the chief astronomer, Takahashi Kageyasu, had given to von Siebold. It was the discovery of this document that led to Takahashi's arrest and von Siebold's deportation.

When von Siebold's illegal possession of this map was exposed in 1828, Takahashi Kageyasu, Inomata Genzaburō, and other *bakufu* officials were arrested and accused of treason. Genboku went to the authorities to declare that he had been an unwitting participant in the conspiracy. He denied knowing the contents of the documents he had given to von Siebold. And when his brother-in-law, Inomata Genzaburō, was convicted of treason and executed, Genboku remained free.[13]

One interpretation of this purge of influential *rangaku* scholar-officials is that the *bakufu*, or a faction within the *bakufu*, wanted to clip the wings of an intellectual elite that showed signs of becoming too independent of the authorities and too closely connected with the Dutch merchant community. Whatever Genboku's involvement in the illicit transfer of the documents may have been, the *bakufu* officials who sought to suppress Japan's *rangaku* scholars probably thought that he was too unimportant for their concern.

Itō Genboku moved to Edo permanently in 1828.[14] He received financial assistance from Aochi Rinsō (1775–1833),[15] a *ranpō* physician he had met at the Tenmondai in 1826, who loaned him the money to set up a medical practice in Edo's Baba district. A year later he moved his practice to Shitaya and opened a private medical school called Shōsendō.[16] Genboku had spent relatively little time on his medical education, but he had taken full advantage of the many connections he had made after leaving Nihiyama. His marriage to the daughter of a senior Dutch interpreter, and his association with von Siebold, however short-lived, provided Genboku with outstanding credentials and gave him immediate standing in Edo's *ranpō* medical community. It was an auspicious beginning.

ŌTSUKI SHUNSAI (1804–1862)

Young men of the same generation as Hino Teisai and Itō Genboku who were born in the Tōhoku region, which comprises Japan's northeastern domains, had virtually no exposure to foreigners of any sort. Even so, those who sought medicine as a career acted very much like their future colleagues in Kyushu. They first sought medical connections within their own communities and used those connections to move to more established centers of medicine. Sendai domain, in particular, produced many *ranpō* physicians, some of whom were leading figures in Edo *rangaku* community.[17]

The medical career of Ōtsuki Shunsai (not related to Ōtsuki Gentaku) proceeded more slowly than the careers of either Hino Teisai or Itō Genboku. Shunsai was born into a low-ranking samurai family in Sendai domain in 1804.[18] The family's intention was for Shunsai, the second of three sons, to be trained and adopted by a physician in a neighboring village. He was sent off at age fifteen to begin his apprenticeship. Had things gone well, Shunsai would have succeeded to the headship of the physician's household, inherited the medical practice of his adoptive father, and become a local physician in Sendai domain. But things did not go well, and within a year Shunsai had returned to his natal home. A few years later, and against his father's wishes, he set off for Edo, where his older brother, who was already in Edo studying Western artillery, offered him financial and logistical assistance.[19]

Ōtsuki Shunsai began his medical career as a servant to Takahashi Shōsai, an Edo physician who practiced *kanpō* medicine, and who eventually accepted Shunsai as a pupil. After several years, Takahashi introduced Shunsai to Tezuka Ryōsen, another Edo physician who also practiced *kanpō* medicine. Tezuka Ryōsen had excellent medical credentials: he had studied under Hara Nanyō, perhaps the most prestigious physician-scholar of Chinese medicine at the beginning of the nineteenth century. Despite his *kanpō* orientation, Tezuka Ryōsen must have had good connections with the *ranpō* medical community, because it was he who introduced Ōtsuki Shunsai to Minato Chōan.

This introduction by a well-known *kanpō* physician to a senior *ranpō* physician suggests that, in Edo as well as in Nagasaki, there was no sharp ideological divide separating *ranpō* and *kanpō* physicians. It also shows that associations and lines of referral between physicians crossed geographical and political boundaries. Domain connections remained important, and referrals to and by influential individuals from one's native place were common and valued, especially in Edo, where domains maintained permanent administrations in which young men could find employment. A good recommendation might secure an office and a stipend in one's domain administration. But Shunsai's introduction to medical training in Edo was made without regard to domain connections. Neither of Ōtsuki Shunsai's physician-teachers was from Sendai. Takahashi Shōsai was from Kawagoe domain, Musashi Province; and Tezuka Ryōsen was from Naganuma domain, Hitachi Province.

Shunsai's introduction to Minato Chōan was important for reasons other than domain solidarity. Minato Chōan was Ōtsuki Shunsai's connection to the Edo *ranpō* and *rangaku* community, which suggests that Shunsai had already openly declared a preference for Western medicine, or that he had been encouraged in that direction by his *kanpō* teachers. However important domain connections might be, if one wished to establish oneself as a *ranpō* physician, introductions to established *ranpō* physicians and to Dutch interpreters were more important than anything else. In Edo, the former connection seems to have been most important; in Nagasaki, the latter connection.

The lateral lines of referral that advanced Ōtsuki Shunsai's interests in Edo suggest that emerging networks were developing outside the more traditional vertical lines of referral. These networks connected physicians across family, domain, and *bakufu* boundaries as individuals began to explore new approaches to medicine. The introduction of Ōtsuki Shunsai to Minato Chōan merged these two referral systems, representing the growing importance of quasi-personal, quasi-professional connections based on common intellectual interests. Given the absence of medical societies and associations that functioned to connect people of similar interests in Europe, this broadening of referral possibilities on the basis of mutual interest was a development of enormous importance.

In his account of the 1826 court journey, von Siebold commented on the geographic diversity of the *ranpō* physicians he met in Japan:

> Just after I arrived in Deshima, in 1823, I came to know some excellent doctors who were staying in Nagasaki. . . . Among them were Minato Chōan, a doctor of high standing in Edo, the young Mima Junzō from Awa, Hirai Kaizō and Oka Kenkai from Mikawa, and many other doctors and scholars from all over Japan.[20]

Minato Chōan had returned to Edo after von Siebold's departure and was appointed to the Translation Bureau at the Tenmondai, where he became an important link between *rangaku* and *ranpō* networks in Edo. He was one of the charter members of the Shōshikai, an eclectic group that brought *bakufu* and domain officials together with physicians, scholars, and artists to discuss the issues of the day. The literal translation of the group's name is "Old Men's Club," but in fact its members were mostly young men. Minato Chōan, who was one of the more senior members, introduced newcomers like Ōtsuki Shunsai to Ito Genboku, Takano Chōei, Koseki San'ei, and other former students of von Siebold who had recently come to Edo from Nagasaki. These men formed the core of the Shōshikai, which for a brief period in the 1830s promoted lateral connections within the Edo community. For Ōtsuki Shunsai, whose formal connections to *ranpō* medicine were in their formative stage, this timely introduction to *ranpō* physicians who had studied with von Siebold in Nagasaki was especially valuable.

In the early 1830s, Shunsai began to study with Adachi Chōshun (1776–1836), a physician and botanist whose early teachers were *kanpō* physicians affiliated with the Igakkan, the Tokugawa *bakufu*'s medical school in Edo. Adachi Chōshun had taken up the study of Western-style obstetrics fairly late in life, but he was the first to translate a book on Western obstetrics into Japanese. Around 1830 he took several recommended *ranpō* physicians as private students, and for a short time, Chōshun's school was a place where men who were working on translations of Western books became acquainted.[21]

Ōtsuki Shunsai studied with Adachi Chōshun until the latter's death in 1836, and then left almost immediately for Nagasaki. By then in his thirties, Shunsai stayed in Nagasaki for four years. There is little record of what he did there, but presumably he studied Dutch, because soon he was translating Dutch medical books. His choice of teacher and books may have been influenced by his older brother, who had studied with Takashima Shūhan, Japan's foremost expert on Western military technology. Shunsai later translated Western medical texts on the treatment of gunshot wounds.[22]

Ōtsuki Shunsai spent almost two decades advancing through the various stages of medical training: local apprentice, urban immigrant, servant, student of *kanpō* and *ranpō* physicians, and, finally, a student of the Dutch language in Nagasaki. Shunsai needed money to pay teachers' fees, to buy books, and to support himself while in Nagasaki. Although he had no regular source of income for many years, he did have a patron, Kanzakiya Genzō. Genzō was an Edo pharmacist who was interested in Western pharmacology, and he supported both Ōtsuki Shunsai and the more famous Takano Chōei, also from Sendai domain. Successful merchants were often patrons of talented individuals, and during the Tokugawa period, merchants were an important source of funding for new initiatives. Genzō became a lifetime supporter of Ōtsuki Shunsai's medical projects.

His teacher, Tezuka Ryōsen, also remained an important sponsor. When Shunsai returned to Edo in 1840, he married Ryōsen's daughter and received an appointment, with stipend, as an official physician to Naganuma domain, the birthplace of his father-in-law. He did not change his surname to Tezuka, probably because Tezuka Ryōsen had a son who would inherit his position. Ōtsuki Shunsai promptly opened a medical practice in Shitaya, within a few city blocks of Itō Genboku's school, initiating what would lead to a lifelong collaboration between these two men.[23] He was thirty-six years old.

SATŌ TAIZEN (1804–1872)

The medical career of Satō Taizen began with the bold strategic moves of his father, Satō Tōsuke, who left his natal village to find employment near Edo.[24] Tōsuke set the pattern for Taizen's brilliant strategies and his rise to prominence. Satō Tōsuke was born in the northern province of Dewa, the eldest son in a poor peasant family. In 1795, at age nineteen, he left home, passing his familial responsibilities as firstborn son to his sister. He found employment with a well-to-do farmer named Tanabe Shōemon in Musashi Province, not far from Edo. Tōsuke was adopted into the Tanabe family as their son and heir in 1802, and he married their adopted daughter, Fuji. Tōsuke took the surname of his adoptive family and became Tanabe Tōsuke. In 1804, Tōsuke and Fuji had a son whom they named Tanabe Shōtarō. This was the future Satō Taizen: he would be known as Tanabe Shōtarō until 1834 when he was thirty years old. He will be referred to here as Satō Taizen, the professional name he took many years later.

In 1805, when Taizen was one year old, Tōsuke had the Tanabe family adopt his infant son, left the Tanabe household to seek employment in Edo, and reclaimed his original surname of Satō. Like adoption and marriage, name changing was an important social and political strategy, although reacquiring one's original surname may have been unusual. How Satō Tōsuke spent the next dozen years is not known, but in 1817 he entered the service of Ina Koretada, a *bakufu* retainer (*hatamoto*) who lived in the Toranomon section of Edo. Tōsuke arranged to bring Taizen, now thirteen, into service with him, and to have him educated with Ina Koretada's young son. Taizen married early, and by 1822 he had two daughters, but he divorced his first wife, who returned to her natal home. The daughters stayed with Taizen, who married the daughter of a *bakufu* retainer in 1826.

Satō Taizen's interest in Western medicine, like Ōtsuki Shunsai's, can be documented from the early 1830s, and the two men followed similar paths. Taizen also became acquainted with Takano Chōei and von Siebold's former students, studied with Adachi Chōshun, attended the meetings of the Shōshi-kai, and became active in the Western-oriented intellectual community developing in Edo at the time. Both men went to Nagasaki in the 1830s. While attending Takano Chōei's school in the Kojimachi district, he met Matsumoto Ryōho, a *bakufu* physician who became Taizen's lifelong friend, associate, and collaborator. These early connections were important. Years later,

Matsumoto Ryōho would adopt Taizen's second son, Ryōjun, later known as Matsumoto Jun.[25]

Taizen remained a servant in the Ina household while pursuing his medical studies in Edo; his second wife and now four children were also residents of the Ina household. In 1834, when Taizen decided to go to Nagasaki, he had to fulfill his service obligations to the Ina family, and he arranged for his brother-in-law to look after his wife and their two sons during his absence. Taizen's two daughters by his first wife were placed in the care of his father, Satō Tōsuke. On the eve of his departure for Nagasaki, Taizen took his mother's surname, Wada, and became Wada Taizen. He was thirty years old.

In 1834, Satō Taizen went to Nagasaki with Hayashi Dōkai, a younger man he had met while studying with Adachi Chōshun. Hayashi Dōkai (1813–1895) had come to Edo in the spring of 1834, and the two men forged an almost immediate alliance, which they would consolidate over many years. Taizen's association with Hayashi Dōkai was an advantageous one. Dōkai was a native of Kokura in Kyushu—the first stop from Nagasaki on the court journey to Edo, and Dōkai had excellent domain connections in Nagasaki. He was able to help Taizen arrange lodging at the home of the Dutch interpreter Suenaga Jinzaemon, who probably was also his teacher. Dōkai entered the school of Ōishi Ryōitsu, a *ranpō* physician with whom he studied the Dutch language and Western medicine.

The two men remained in Nagasaki for three years. Despite the remarkable documentation of these travel and accommodation details, it is not at all clear how they spent their time in Nagasaki. Their living arrangements and undated scholarly output suggest that they spent their time translating Dutch medical texts.[26] The only evidence that either of them formally studied Western medicine while residing in Nagasaki is the fact that Hayashi Dōkai was enrolled in the school of the *ranpō* physician Ōishi Ryōitsu.

The 1830s were not a good time to study *ranpō* medicine in Nagasaki, and those who were there at that time had a very different experience than those who had studied in Nagasaki in the 1820s. Following von Siebold's deportation, Dutch physicians no longer came to Dejima, and Japanese physicians were forbidden to have any direct contact with the Dutch.[27] Study in Nagasaki seems to have been an exercise in establishing good credentials and contacts. Physicians who went to Nagasaki after 1830 probably educated

themselves by translating Western medical books under the guidance of a
Nagasaki interpreter or someone who knew Dutch. While this might have
been accomplished just as well in Edo, the Nagasaki experience was highly
valued, and Nagasaki was still the only place where Dutch medical books
could enter Japan. The Nagasaki experience also gave men who had been
busy practicing medicine in Edo time to work on translations.

Satō (Wada) Taizen and Hayashi Dōkai returned to Edo in 1838, and Taizen opened a medical practice and school. He called his school Wada-juku
but reclaimed his father's original surname, Satō, at that time. Thereafter he
was known as Satō Taizen. Hayashi Dōkai lived with the Taizen's family in
Edo for three years, and in 1841 Taizen sent him back to Nagasaki for further
study. When Dōkai returned to Edo in 1843 he became the head of Wada-
juku, took over Taizen's medical practice, and married Taizen's eldest daughter. Taizen's second son, Ryōjun, now age five, was put in the care of his
daughter and new son-in-law, Hayashi Dōkai.[28]

Having put his affairs in order in this way, Satō Taizen moved on. In 1843,
he left Edo to enter the service of Hotta Masayoshi, Lord of Sakura domain.
Sakura was a domain to the east of Edo in today's Chiba Prefecture. Taizen
had excellent reasons for moving to Sakura.[29] Hotta Masayoshi was a rising
star in national politics during the 1840s. A decade earlier, he had begun to
build a Western studies center in Sakura, and in 1835 he had founded a domain medical school. From the outset, the school curriculum included the
study of Western medicine: kanpō medicine was taught on odd-numbered
days and ranpō medicine on even-numbered days.[30] During the late 1830s and
early 1840s, Hotta sent domain physicians to Nagasaki to study Western-
style medicine, and they returned to Sakura to teach what they had learned.
The school attracted established physicians, like Mitsukuri Genpo, a respected ranpō physician and translator of Dutch books.

Hotta Masayoshi's invitation to Satō Taizen to inaugurate and direct a new
Western-style medical academy in Sakura domain was an unusual opportunity. The school was called Juntendō: it was Japan's first medical school dedicated solely to the teaching and practice of Western medicine and surgery.[31]
Juntendō became a training center for surgeons who began to perform new
surgical techniques.[32] In 1847, when Taizen's son Ryōjun became fifteen, he
moved from Edo to Sakura to begin his training in Western-style medicine
and surgery.

OGATA KŌAN (1810–1863)

Ogata Kōan is the best known of the seven *ranpō* physician-scholars.[33] He was born in 1810 in Ashimori, Bitchū Province (now part of the city of Okayama), the third son of the samurai Saeki Sezaemon. As a child he was called Seinosuke, and he became Ogata Kōan only after many name changes. The many accounts of Kōan's exemplary life record even the most minor events; however, there is no mention of his youth or early education. His life seems to begin in 1825 when he reached the age of fourteen. As the third son, Kōan was not entitled to any hereditary office or stipend, and the time had come to prepare for his future.[34]

Kōan's options may have been better than those of younger sons born to peasant households, but his samurai rank actually placed some restrictions on the possibilities open to him. It was not acceptable for him to take off on his own, or to work as a farmer or servant, as Satō Tōsuke did, because doing so would have disgraced his family. Decisions about what to do and how to do it had to be appropriate to his samurai status. For this reason, perhaps, small decisions were carefully recorded for posterity in the family's household records. They tell us, for example, that at his coming of age ceremony, Kōan added a character from his father's name to his own childhood name, and that three months later he chose an entirely different name.[35] To avoid confusion, he will be referred to here as Ogata Kōan, the professional name he chose in 1836 when he was twenty-five.

In 1825, Kōan accompanied his father on a business trip to Osaka. When they returned to Ashimori the following year, Kōan wrote a deferential letter to his parents explaining that he was unsuited to the life of a samurai because he was not physically strong. The letter states his wish to relinquish his samurai status, become a physician, and work to relieve the suffering of the sick. He claimed to have entertained this idea for three years. A photograph of this private, personal letter to his parents, renouncing his samurai status, is often exhibited in Kōan's biographies.[36] The preservation of this letter, documenting compelling reasons for Kōan's request for a change of status, was undoubtedly important to his family as well as his domain lord.

The trip to Osaka the previous year may have been an official business trip, but subsequent events make it apparent that father and son went together to arrange for Kōan to enter an appropriate school. He entered the private academy of Naka Ten'yū (1783–1835) in Osaka in the summer of 1826. There is no indication that he had any prior exposure to *kanpō* medicine, or for that matter to any education at all, but clearly Ogata Kōan could read and write and had probably been educated in the Chinese classics. The choice of Naka Ten'yū's school, Shishisai-juku in Osaka, strongly suggests that he had contemplated a commitment to Western medicine for some time, and that the trip to Osaka soon after Kōan became of age was but the first overt step in a well-conceived plan.

Why Ogata Kōan chose a school dedicated to Dutch learning and *ranpō* medicine rather than *kanpō* medicine is not clear. *Rangaku* studies were flourishing in Osaka in the 1820s, and a career in Western medicine may have seemed a more promising opportunity for a younger son with few prospects. If so, Naka Ten'yū's school was an excellent place to begin. Naka Ten'yū was not a physician, and his school might seem an odd choice for a young man who had just announced his intention to become a physician. However, Ten'yū was one of Osaka's foremost *rangaku* scholars, he had strong connections with scholar-physicians in both Edo and Nagasaki, and he was considered the best teacher of the Dutch language in the Kansai region.

Naka Ten'yū (1783–1835) was born in Kyoto, but he had studied in Edo with Ōtsuki Gentaku, spent a brief period in Nagasaki, and then studied with prominent *rangaku* scholars in the Kansai area. He was best known for his translations of Dutch books on astronomy.[37] Kōan studied at Ten'yū's school for four years and became an excellent Dutch scholar and translator. By the time he had finished his studies in Osaka, Ogata Kōan was already regarded as a future leader of *rangaku* studies.[38]

In the spring of 1830, Ogata Kōan went to Edo and entered Nisshūdō, Tsuboi Shindō's school in Edo's Fukagawa district. Tsuboi Shindō (1795–1848) *was* a physician, and he had been teaching *ranpō* medicine in Edo for about ten years. Shindō had studied Chinese and Chinese-style medicine before becoming interested in Western medicine. He had then become a student of Udagawa Genshin, the prolific translator of Western medical texts. Tsuboi Shindō had not gone to Nagasaki to study, but he became close friends with both Itō Genboku and Totsuka Seika, who had studied with von Siebold. During the 1830s, these three physicians—Shindō, Genboku, and Seikai—were widely known in Edo as "the three Dutch scholars." Ogata Kōan's affiliation with Tsuboi Shindō connected him to the Edo network of established *ranpō* physicians, as well as newcomers from all over Japan who came to study in Edo. It was Shindō who introduced Kōan to the ailing Udagawa Genshin, so that Kōan could work with him on some translations. There could be no clearer indication that Ogata Kōan had earned his teacher's favor.

Unlike Ōtsuki Shunsai, also of samurai rank, Ogata Kōan made no false starts. He entered the best schools at a young age and he received the finest training in Dutch and in *ranpō* medicine that was available at the time. His greatest difficulty seems to have been choosing a name, which he changed again several times while in Edo.[39]

Two of his teachers died in 1835, and that year became a year of transition for Ogata Kōan. When Udagawa Genshin died in Edo at the beginning of 1835, Kōan returned home to Ashimori.[40] A month later, he received word of Naka Ten'yū's death, and he went almost immediately to Osaka.[41] He remained in Osaka for about a year, lecturing and teaching Dutch to the students at Ten'yū's school. Then, in early 1836, with Naka Ten'yū's young son in tow, Kōan set off for Nagasaki to begin the final stage of his preparation for a career devoted to *ranpō* medicine. It was at this point that he changed his name, permanently, to Ogata Kōan.

Kōan returned to Osaka in 1838 and opened his private academy, Tekitekisai-juku (better known as Tekijuku), which would establish his reputation as Japan's foremost *ranpō* scholar-physician. He married a physician's daughter named Yae, age fourteen, the same year. For the next twenty-five years, Ogata Kōan would remain in Osaka working as a physician, a teacher of the Dutch language, and a prolific translator of Western medical books. Tekijuku would become a truly national school that promoted cross-regional and cross-class connections for the first time.[42] Kōan had devoted many years to developing his Dutch language skills, and at Tekijuku he focused on teaching students those same skills. Many of the students who came to Tekijuku used these skills to study subjects other than medicine. His most famous student, Nagayo Sensai, the Meiji government's first Director of Public Health, claimed that whatever one's interest, the most important activity at Tekijuku was translating Dutch texts.[43]

KUWATA RYŪSAI (1811–1868)

Kuwata Ryūsai was the youngest of the seven physicians. He began his life as Muramatsu Kiuemon in Echigo Province in 1811, the second son of a father of low samurai rank.[44] His samurai status allowed him to attend his domain school, and he developed an early interest in medicine. He next attended the domain medical school, where he studied the standard Chinese and Japanese medical texts, and possibly he learned about Western medicine from Dutch medical books in the medical school library. When he expressed an interest in going to Edo to study *ranpō* medicine, his father wrote to his former horseback-riding instructor in Edo to arrange lodging for his son in Edo's Fukagawa district. Kiuemon went to Edo in 1826 and again in 1829, and he enrolled in Tsuboi Shindō's school, where Ogata Kōan must also have been studying at the time.

Muramatsu Kiuemon apparently did well enough to secure an introduction to Kuwata Genshin, an Edo *kanpō* physician who specialized in children's diseases. Kuwata Genshin was already performing Western-style variolation, and he had written and published a book on variolation in 1814. Kiuemon assisted Kuwata Genshin in his pediatric medical practice until 1841, when Genshin adopted him as his son and heir. At the age of thirty, Muramatsu Kiuemon became Kuwata Ryūsai. Ryūsai never studied in Nagasaki, and probably he was never proficient in Dutch, but perhaps because of his adoptive father's early commitment to variolation and his experiences treating children with smallpox, Kuwata Ryūsai's personal contribution to the transmission of Jennerian vaccination in Japan would be outstanding.

KASAHARA HAKUŌ (1809–1880)

The last of the seven physicians to be considered here is Kasahara Hakuō. He was born Kasahara Ryūsaku in 1809, in a small village near the city of Fukui, in Echizen Province on the Japan Sea.[45] Unlike the other six men, Ryūsaku was a *kanpō* physician's son, and his entry into the world of *ranpō* medicine followed a quite different trajectory. It was Ryūsaku's father, Kasahara Ryūsai, who had made the transition from farming to medicine and secured an appointment as an official physician of Fukui domain. This office entitled his son to a classical education and medical training at the Fukui domain school. Ryūsaku first studied the Chinese classics with a local Confucian scholar. Beginning at age fifteen, he studied *kanpō* medicine at the Fukui domain school for five years. He then went to Edo, where he studied *kanpō* medicine for another three years.

This vague chronology places Kasahara Ryūsaku in Edo between 1829 and

1832, when practicing *ranpō* physicians were just beginning to form a broader, and more active, intellectual community in Edo. There is no evidence that Ryūsaku was associated with this community or that he became acquainted with any of the officials, scholars, physicians, and vaccination advocates with whom he would later collaborate. Ryūsaku had gone to Edo to augment his Chinese-style medical education in the capital, and neither his interests nor his affiliations would necessarily have intersected with any of the other six physicians at this time. Kasahara Ryūsaku returned to Echizen in 1832 and set up a practice in *kanpō* medicine in the city of Fukui.

Whether Ryūsaku was influenced by his experiences in Edo in some way, or whether he became dissatisfied after he returned to Fukui, he experienced some important shift in his thinking during his late twenties. He next appears in Kyoto in the mid-1830s as a student of Hino Teisai, the first physician discussed above. Hino Teisai provides a clear link between Kasahara Ryūsaku and Western medicine, but it is unclear how this connection developed. Ryūsaku never studied Dutch in Nagasaki—perhaps a second-generation physician with a secure livelihood waiting for him in Fukui did not need Dutch credentials. Possibly he knew very little Dutch, but there is no doubt that Hino Teisai transmitted his own commitment to Western medicine, and to vaccination in particular, to the younger man. Ryūsaku returned to Fukui a devoted advocate of Western medicine and an avid proponent of vaccination. He may have received a more direct injection of enthusiasm for Western medicine from Teisai than would have been possible in Nagasaki during the bleak period after von Siebold's departure.

Whatever Ryūsaku's educational deficiencies, he demonstrated his support for vaccination by changing his name to Hakuō. The character for *haku* was intended to mimic the sound "vacc" in the word "vaccine," thus Hakuō's new name was a personal and public statement of his commitment to vaccination. Kasahara Hakuō would not move to Edo until the end of his life, but he insured the continuation of his own medical lineage, now devoted to *ranpō* not *kanpō* medicine, by adopting his younger brother and sending him to study with Ogata Kōan at Tekijuku.

*   *   *

By now it should be apparent that there was a great deal more to becoming a *ranpō* physician than studying Western-style medicine. Each of the physicians discussed above employed strategies that linked merit to occupation and inheritance. Medicine may have been a hereditary occupation that passed from father to son, but we can see that adoption and marriage strategies provided a way of establishing new medical linkages, as well as continuing an established family line and occupation. Both strategies rewarded talent and created opportunities while upholding the stability of families, households, property, and status over many generations. They also circumvented the rigid Tokugawa class system, which was designed to keep everyone in his allotted place.

The possibility of a beneficial adoption gave talented young men an incentive to seek opportunity in fields that interested them and to treat their teachers and benefactors well. Upward mobility requires risk taking, but it could not have been clear in the 1830s that *ranpō* medicine would offer a promising future. In the short term, it must have seemed a treacherous path to follow. The arrest and execution of von Siebold's Japanese associates in 1829 was the first serious purge of Western learning scholars, but it would not be the last. A decade later another *bakufu* purge ended with the deaths or suicides of several more of von Siebold's students and members of the Shōshikai in Edo.[46]

For those who survived, becoming a *ranpō* physician required an enormous personal transformation: a change of social status and social space; often several changes in one's name, household, and geographic location; and an itinerant way of life and uncertain future for long periods. The idea of a self-made man did not exist: each individual, however ambitious or talented, had to depend heavily on the influence and assistance of others.

By 1840, all seven physicians had finished their formal medical education and were practicing medicine in one of Japan's major cities or towns. Itō Genboku, Ōtsuki Shunsai, Kuwata Ryūsai, and Satō Taizen were in Edo; Hino Teisai was in Kyoto; Ogata Kōan was in Osaka; and Kasahara Hakuō was in Fukui. Several of them had founded their own Western-style medical schools: Hino Teisai's school in Kyoto, Ogata Kōan's Tekijuku in Osaka, and Itō Genboku's Shōsendō and Satō Taizen's Wada-juku in Edo. In 1843, Satō Taizen would move to Sakura to found Juntendō, but his former school, Wada-juku, continued under the direction of his son-in-law, Hayashi Dōkai. These central places, with Nagasaki, formed the major geographical nodes of a developing *ranpō* physicians' network.

The student register at Ogata Kōan's Tekijuku lists the names of 636 students from forty-five domains who studied there; a similar register from Itō Genboku's Shosendō lists 403 names from forty-four domains.[47] Most of the students came from domains in southwestern and northeastern Japan, and these schools clearly functioned as magnet institutions where physicians interested in Western-style medicine might become acquainted. Quite a few students appear on the registers of more than one school, indicating the itinerant nature of Western-style medical education in the late Tokugawa period. These and other private medical schools founded to promote Western-style medicine were enormously important after 1830 in disseminating medical knowledge to a larger, younger, and more diverse audience. Richard Rubinger's excellent work on several of these schools documents their importance and influence in the late Tokugawa and early Meiji periods.[48] By the mid-nineteenth century, these schools had greatly expanded the number of physicians who would promote vaccination when cowpox vaccine became available.

TRANSLATION

Translating Western medical texts was especially important to the construction of *ranpō* networks. Table 5.2 lists the publication years and topics of European medical books translated in the 1830s and 1840s by five of the seven physicians discussed above. Most remarkable is the speed with which recently published European medical texts were reaching Japan. Many of these books had been written only a short time before by German academic physicians who held prestigious faculty positions in European universities. They were quickly translated into Dutch and sent off to Japan. This suggests that a specialized market for Dutch medical books had developed in Japan, and that Nagasaki interpreters were ordering books that they would then sell to Japanese booksellers and special clients. Before the 1820s, *rangaku* scholars, as often as not, had translated European books written a century or so earlier. Although it is rarely possible to know exactly when particular books were imported and translated, because few of these translations were published at the time, it is quite clear that *ranpō* physicians were translating the writings of European contemporaries. The marked increase in translations of recent medical works is impressive, especially given the fact that government suppression of Western scholarship was increasing during this period.

Was von Siebold a catalyst for this upsurge of interest in and translation of German medical books? It is reasonable to think so. During the 1820s, von Siebold had introduced his students at Narutaki to the writings of prominent,

TABLE 5.2

Publication years of European medical books translated by Ranpō *physicians*

Japanese Translator European Author (birth/death years)	Original Publication Year (Language)	Dutch Publication Year	Main Topics/Types of Books Translated	Japanese Translation/ Publication Year
Hino Teisai				
Dzondi, K.H. (1770–1835)	1826 (German)	1827	Syphilis	?/X
Itō Genboku				
I. R. Bischoff (1784–1835)	1823–1825 (German)	1826–1828	Internal medicine	?/1835–1858
A. Moll/C. Eldik (1786–1843/ 1791–1857)		1822–1856	Dutch medical journal	1842–1843/X
C. W. Hufeland (1762–1836)	1836 (German)	1838	Vaccination	?/X
Ōtsuki Shunsai				
M. J. von Chelius (1794–1876)	1831	1830–1832	Gunshot wounds	1854/1854
G. F. Most (1794–1845)	(German) 1833 (German)	1835–1839	"	1854/1854
Satō Taizen				
M.J. von Chelius (1794–1876)	1831 (German)	1830–1832	Bone-setting	1837–1838/X
C. W. Hufeland (1762–1836)	1798 (German)	1802	Smallpox case histories	1837–1838/X
G. F. Most (1794–1845)	1833 (German)	1835–1839	Eye diseases Vaccination	?/X
Ogata Kōan				
C. W. Hufeland (1762–1836)	1836 (German)	1837–1838	Pathology Vaccination	?/1849
A. Moll/C. Eldik (1786–1843/ 1791–1857)	1822–1856 (Dutch)	1822–1856	Dutch medical journal	1842–1843/X
G. F. Most (1794–1843)	1833 (German)	1835–1839	Encyclopedia	1838/X
T. Schwencke (1693–1767)	1753 (German)	1753	Prescriptions	1838/X
J. W. H. Conradi (1780–1861)	1826–1828 (German)	1832–1837	Articles on Cholera	1858/1858
G. F. Most (1794–1876)	1833 (German)	1835–1839	"	1858/1858
C. Canstatt (1807–1850)	1841–1847 (German)	1843–1854	"	1858/1858

Source: Miyashita, Saburō. "A bibliography of the Dutch medical books translated into Japanese." *Archives internationales d'histoire des sciences* 25, no. 96 (1975): 8–72.

? = Translation year unknown

X = Unpublished manuscript

contemporary German physicians such as C. W. Hufeland, and he had them translate selections from these books.[49] Whether he brought these books with him or whether they were imported later is not clear, but the fact that his students became heavily involved in the translation of German medical books after von Siebold's departure in 1829 suggests that he made them aware of the importance of certain writers. Thirteen of von Siebold's students were responsible for sixty-five different translations; two of his students, Takano Chōei and Kō Ryōsai, translated thirty-five books between them.[50]

Translations by practicing physicians were private translations, and they differed from the translations by scholars who worked under *bakufu* or domain sponsorship. Whereas the translations of the Udagawa and other elite medical lineages focused on what would have been regarded as the basic sciences in the West—physics, chemistry, anatomy, pathology, botany, zoology, and pharmacology—the translations of practicing physicians with patients to treat and students and apprentices to train were interested in practical solutions to everyday medical problems.[51] Hino Teisai, for example, translated a book on syphilis; Ōtsuki Shunsai, a book on gunshot wounds; Ogata Kōan, information about eye diseases and cholera; and Itō Genboku and Satō Taizen translated books about approaches to specific medical and surgical problems. The European physicians whose writings they translated had a similar purpose: they, too, were teaching students, documenting their own experiences, and recommending therapies to colleagues.

One of the most influential European physicians at the time was Christoph Wilhelm Hufeland (1762–1836), a German physician of international reputation whose writings were popular in Europe for most of the nineteenth century. It is not difficult to understand why Hufeland's writings appealed to Japan's *ranpō* physicians. Hufeland wrote for his fellow medical practitioners, and his books covered many fields of medicine. His *Enchiridion medicum*, based on fifty years of medical experience, was first published in Berlin in 1836, the year of his death.[52] This small, comprehensive text is a compendium of "Maxims and General Rules for Beginning Practitioners." A section on "Practice" is divided into thirteen classes of medicine, and the "Disease" class is subdivided into many ailments known at the time.

Enchiridion medicum was translated into many European languages: Dutch editions were published in 1837 and 1838; a French edition in 1838; Italian in 1856; and English editions, in England and the United States, at least five times between 1842 and 1855. Hufeland was already known in Japan when

Enchiridion medicum was published in Germany. Tsuboi Shindō and Udagawa Yōan were translating Hufeland's earlier writings when they began to study with Ogata Kōan in the early 1830s. A Dutch edition of *Enchiridon medicum* made its way quickly to Japan, and Japanese translations were underway by the late 1830s.

At least twelve Japanese physicians translated various sections of *Enchiridion medicum*.[53] Ogata Kōan's translation, *Hu-shi keiken ikun* (*Mr. Hu's {Hufeland's} Medical Experience*) is one of the famous translations of the Edo period. It is based on the second Dutch edition of 1838 and covers all the "Practice" sections.[54] Kōan referred to this long-term project as *Ikun*. By 1842, he had a first draft in hand, which he sent to Tsuboi Shindō, his former teacher in Edo, for advice and comments. *Ikun* was not published until 1857, but Kōan's correspondence shows that he frequently discussed this lengthy translation with his students and associates long before that.[55]

Georg Frederick Most (1794–1845) was another German physician whose writings appealed to *ranpō* physicians. The format of his *Encyklopädie* on medical and surgical practice made it possible for them to find short entries and basic information about a wide range of topics.[56] Satō Taizen, Hayashi Dōkai, Ōtsuki Shunsai, Ogata Kōan, and Tsuboi Shindō, plus two of von Siebold's students, Itō Keisuke and Takenouchi Gendō, all consulted Most's *Encyklopädie* and translated excerpts from it. These translations covered Most's entries on beriberi, bubonic plague, cholera, cancer, diabetes, eye diseases, stroke, venereal disease, and vaccination.

Miyashita Saburō has identified 473 Japanese translations from 189 different Dutch medical books extant in libraries, archives, and private collections in Japan today.[57] The titles of these Japanese translations often have little relationship to the original title or to the topic under consideration. It seems to have been more important to identify the European authors. Titles frequently used the author's surname (or first syllable of the surname) in the title of the translation: C. W. Hufeland became Hu-shi (Mr. Hu), as in *Hu-shi keiken ikun* (*Mr. Hu's Medical Experience*). G. F. Most became Mosuto-shi (Mr. Mosuto); and M. J. Chelius became Che-shi (Mr. Che). At first, these Western names were written phonetically using *katakana,* a script for foreign words. Later these names were assigned Chinese characters, or *kanji,* which makes deciphering these names in Japanese sources even more difficult.

In addition to these individual private translations, there was a brief collaborative effort to produce Japan's first medical journal, *Taisei meii-ikō* (*Jour-*

nal of Articles by Western Physicians). The journal was edited and published by Mitsukuri Genpo between 1836 and 1843.[58] It includes translations of sixteen articles that had been published in the Dutch journal *Practisch tijdschrift voor de geneeskunde* (1822–1856), edited by Anthonij Moll and Cornelis van Eldik.[59] Udagawa Yōan wrote a preface for the first volume in 1836, and Tsuboi Shindō a preface for the second volume. Itō Genboku, Ōtsuki Shunsai, Hayashi Dōkai, Ogata Kōan, and Aoki Kenzō, another student of von Siebold's, all contributed to this journal.[60] They referred to their translations as "The First-hand Experiences of Two Physicians: Eldik and Moll," indicating that they were well aware of the provenance of the journal. The collaboration of these physicians in publishing a Japanese medical journal suggests that copies of *Practisch tijdschrift* were brought to Japan and circulated among the Edo physicians, and that professional, collaborative links existed between the translators of Dutch medical texts. By the end of the Tokugawa period, Japan's *ranpō* physicians had created a body of medical literature in Japanese based on a large number of translations from Dutch medical books.

How to assess the impact of all these medical translations? Western medical therapies had few advantages over Japanese medicine in the 1830s and 1840s. Therapies, such as bleeding and purging, commonly used to treat medical problems in the West, were deleterious to health and healing, and Japanese medical practice may well have been more benign, if not more effective. Pharmacology was as advanced in Japan, as in Europe, where medicinal plants still played a major role in treatment, although they used them differently. This may explain why Japanese and Dutch Factory physicians were interested in sharing and comparing botanical knowledge and plants.[61] Although surgery was definitely more advanced in the West, it was a limited option everywhere before the advent of anesthesia.

Given the limitations of Western medicine, the impact of Japanese translations of Dutch medical writings on contemporary Japanese medical practice must have been fairly limited. However, these translations were extraordinarily important in creating a generation of medical scholars with a common knowledge base and intellectual connections to European physicians. The translations prompted experimentation and discussion of different medical approaches among Japanese physicians; they encouraged collaboration and the copying and sharing of texts. Perhaps most important of all, they promoted foreign-language learning skills, which made it possible for Japanese scholars to read and communicate in a written language not based on the Chinese writing system. While much has been made of the limited usefulness of the Dutch language in the mid-nineteenth-century world, Dutch was an extremely useful bridge to languages that used a Western alphabet. The transmission of medical and other foreign knowledge through the medium of the Dutch language was of no small consequence to those who would become Japan's leaders, many of whom were physicians, after the fall of the Tokugawa shogunate. With the discovery of the germ theory of disease in the 1880s, European scientific medicine would surge ahead of other medical approaches, and Japanese physicians were well positioned to contribute to the host of medical discoveries that followed.

If we accept that there were few differences in the efficacy of general medical treatment in Japan, Europe, and elsewhere during the early nineteenth century, we must also acknowledge the notable exception of Jennerian vaccination, which was being used throughout the world to immunize children against smallpox. Wherever national vaccination programs were in place, smallpox death rates were falling. Regardless of whether Japanese physicians had learned about vaccination from Europeans resident in Japan or from Chinese, European, or Japanese books, they saw vaccination as an obvious answer to the age-old problem of smallpox. With no obvious way to obtain cowpox vaccine, some Japanese physicians began to experiment with various combinations of Chinese-style and Turkish-style variolation.

VARIOLATION

As discussed in Chapter 1, toward the end of the eighteenth century, a few Japanese physicians began to show an interest in both Chinese- and Western-style variolation. In Kyushu during the 1790s, Ogata Shunsaku performed and wrote about Chinese-style variolation, and A. L. Keller demonstrated Western-style inoculation. A decade later, the pediatrician Kuwata Genshin began using Western-style variolation in Edo. He published a book about this method in 1814, and later taught the method to his adopted son, Kuwata Ryūsai. Ōtsuki Gentaku published a book describing Keller's method of variolation in 1816.

By the 1830s, a Japanese-Dutch mixed method of variolation was developing. The physician made a powder from the scabs of patients who had been variolated, a small wound was made in a child's arm, and the powder was placed in the wound. This method, using human smallpox virus, with lymph or scabs, was called *jintō shutō*. As one physician wrote, "After a day a pock emerged, and if pocks produced in this way are compared with a pock from a natural case of smallpox, there were few serious cases. I used this method of variolation on my three younger brothers and one younger sister."[62]

Satō Taizen was experimenting with smallpox variolation in Edo before he went to Nagasaki in 1835. Taizen's second son, Ryōjun (Matsumoto Jun), later wrote about being inoculated at age three:

> My father, Satō Taizen-sensei, had read Conradi's book on medical treatment and he was impressed. As the fourth child, I was the first to be inoculated.[63] Many doctors did this secretly, knowing its great advantage, and they devoted themselves to explaining it to the public. Gradually it came to be widely practiced.[64]

Upon his return from Nagasaki, Taizen wrote a treatise in which he reviewed the writings of several European physicians on variolation, among which were books by C. W. Hufeland, J. A. Water, G. F. Most, J. W. H. Conradi, and others. His treatise, "Tōka shussei," is not a translation but a research paper in which Taizen reviewed twenty-three cases of inoculation cited in European texts and compared his own experiences with those of the European doctors.[65] Taizen also translated the entry on vaccination in G. F. Most's *Encyklopädie* sometime after 1839. He called it "Mosuto's gyūtō hen" ("Most on Cowpox").

Itō Genboku also was experimenting with *jintō shutō* by the 1840s. Genboku was a close friend of Ōtsuki Bankei, whose father, Ōtsuki Gentaku, had discussed variolation techniques with Keller and published a Japanese translation of Lorenz Heister's "On Variolation" in 1816.[66] When Bankei's eldest son died of smallpox during a severe epidemic in 1841, Bankei was reminded of his father's early interest in variolation, and he discussed the possibility of inoculating his other children with Itō Genboku. Although many people were afraid to have their children inoculated with human pox, the two men decided to inoculate Bankei's four younger children, and they had an excellent result. Later, during an epidemic in 1846, Genboku inoculated the daughter of the Sendai *daimyō*. He reported that the inoculation produced a mild case of smallpox with only three small scars.[67]

These details suggest that there was considerable resistance to inoculation with smallpox virus, and that the technique was used primarily during epidemics when the risk of dying from natural smallpox was high. Moreover, as the few accounts cited here suggest, inoculation was practiced in secret and usually confined to family members and trusted friends. The disease of smallpox could not be contained in this fashion.

VACCINATION

The difficulties associated with variolation may have convinced Japanese physicians that the time had come to launch a concerted effort to import cowpox vaccine. The most recent attempt, in 1839, to bring fresh lymph from Holland by way of Batavia had failed.[68] A new approach to the problem was clearly needed. In the 1840s, several physicians tried to persuade their domain lords (*daimyō*) to find a way to import cowpox vaccine. Although they were unable to demonstrate the benefits and safety of vaccination, the medical knowledge they had gained over the previous two decades enabled them to make a compelling case that vaccination was the most effective way to prevent smallpox—and that it was not dangerous. Their translations of current European texts that supported the superiority of vaccination, along with their own experiences with variolation, had given them the confidence they needed to try to gain the support of their domain lords.

C. W. Hufeland, for example, had published a clear opinion on the superiority of vaccination. Hufeland had supported variolation before Jenner published his *Inquiry*, but he quickly shifted his support to vaccination in articles he published in *Journal der praktischen Heilkunde*, a journal he edited.[69] And in *Enchiridion medicum,* he left no doubt that he advocated vaccination as the best way to prevent smallpox:

> Vaccination is one of the greatest and most salutary discoveries of modern times. Protection from small pox may be attained in two different ways; either by avoiding the virus, separation; or by annihilating the susceptibility to it. The first is totally impracticable on account of the intercourse of mankind, and the impossibility there is to avoid infected substances, which are so without our being able to perceive it. Therefore there remains only the second protective method, annihilation of the susceptibility. An endeavor to attain this end was made by the artificial inoculation of the small pox itself; for this disease generally has the peculiarity of annihilating for ever a future susceptibility, and experience had taught that artificial infection, the patient being properly prepared, was less dangerous than the natural one. But there

remained still some danger (one case in five hundred), besides a perpetuation of the variolous virus. . . . Edward Jenner of England, made the first trial of vaccinating the human species, carrying in this way the discovery into practical use. It will easily be conceived how superiour this vaccination is to the inoculation of human small pox, since there is never any danger from it, and man escapes a formidable malady by undergoing an insignificant, often a scarcely perceptible cutaneous affection, and by which he escapes a most hideous disfiguration. Vaccination has since been spread, not alone throughout Europe, but throughout the world, and in many countries it is enforced by legal enactments, which at the same time strictly prohibit the inoculation of human small pox[70]

Properly administered, Hufeland claimed, "This artificial disease [cowpox] requires no medical treatment. The vaccinated may be allowed to continue their customary mode of living."[71] *Ranpō* physicians looking for a testimonial needed to look no further for authoritative backing: variolation might provide effective immunization, but vaccination was better and safer for everyone concerned. But these physicians also knew that Chinese physicians had found cowpox scabs to be less fragile and more easily stored than cowpox lymph; and they knew from their own experiences with variolation that the smallpox virus also remained viable for longer periods when stored as scabs. Might it not be worthwhile to try to transmit live cowpox virus, stored as scabs, from Batavia to Nagasaki?

It took several years to convince the Dutch, who were accustomed to performing vaccination with cowpox lymph, to send the virus as cowpox scabs. In the 1840s, pressure to import cowpox vaccine came from all sides. Hotta Masayoshi, the Lord of Sakura domain and Satō Taizen's patron and employer, may have been the first, in 1843, to formally request that cowpox vaccine be sent to Japan from Batavia in the form of scabs: "Demanded for 1844 by the Second Chancellor, Hotta Settsu no Kami Sama [Hotta Masayoshi]: *5 korst van koepokken voor vacsine* (5 crusts of cowpox for vaccine)."[72] Hotta's request is found in a list of requests submitted that year to the Dutch merchants at Dejima by Japan's highest-ranking officials.

Itō Genboku and Ōtsuki Shunsai both wrote to the authorities in Nagasaki to try again to obtain vaccine from Batavia, and in 1847, Genboku sent a petition asking the assistance of his domain lord, Nabeshima Naomasa, the Saga *daimyō*.[73] Naomasa asked the Dutch merchants to bring cowpox vaccine in 1848, but once again it was no longer viable when it arrived in Nagasaki. In

1848, Narabayashi Sōken repeated Hotta Masayoshi's request that the Dutch send the vaccine virus in the form of crusts the following year.

While these requests went forward, Kasahara Hakuō in Fukui was taking a different tack. Hakuō recently had read *Intō shinpō zensho,* the Japanese translation of *Yin dou lue* (*Outline on Guiding Smallpox*) published in China in 1817. He had been startled to learn that the Chinese had been practicing vaccination for almost half a century. A different solution seemed obvious: why not import cowpox vaccine from China? Hakuō asked his domain lord, Matsudaira Yoshinaga (Keiei), to petition the *bakufu* for permission to import vaccine from China. Yoshinaga, a known supporter of Western studies, complied, submitting petitions in 1847 and again in 1848. This second petition was approved by the Tokugawa Rōjū, Abe Masahiro, who ordered the Governor of Nagasaki to import cowpox vaccine from China.[74]

It is not entirely clear that either *bakufu* or domain permission was needed to import the vaccine virus. Permission had not been requested when cowpox lymph was sent to Nagasaki in the 1820s. But official opposition to Western-style medicine and the activities of *ranpō* physicians had grown since the 1820s, and the political climate for *ranpō* physicians had become far more dangerous. In 1849, the Igakkan issued a ban against the importation of Western books and the practice of Western medicine (with the exception of surgery and ophthalmology). In this climate, obtaining *bakufu* approval and the backing of important domain lords to import cowpox vaccine must have seemed wise.

If the ban against the practice of Western medicine was intended to dissuade its practitioners, it failed. Ironically, in 1849, Japanese-Dutch collaborative efforts to import cowpox vaccine finally produced results.

SIX

The Vaccinators

On August 11, 1849, the *Stad Dordrecht* arrived at the port of Nagasaki. Batavia had honored Narabayashi Sōken's request to send cowpox matter in the form of scabs.[1] The Director of Health at Batavia had attended to it himself and seen that both *lympha* and *pokroven* had been prepared for the voyage to Japan. Upon their arrival in Nagasaki, both forms of the virus were given to the Factory physician, Otto Mohnike. Three days later, Opperhoofd Joseph Henrij Levyssohn wrote the following report in the *Dagregister*:

> 14 August. Today Dr. Mohnike used the cowpox material that recently arrived from Batavia to vaccinate three Japanese children. According to a message from the *onderrapporteur*, the Governor of Nagasaki has granted permission for a young Japanese doctor to enter Deshima daily to be instructed by Dr. Mohnike.[2]

Two of the three children Mohnike vaccinated were children of Nagasaki interpreters; the third was Narabayashi Sōken's third son, Kensaburō. Acting on instructions from his domain lord, Nabeshima Naomasa, Narabayashi

Sōken had personally accompanied the children to the Dutch Factory doctor to be vaccinated.[3]

Otto Mohnike vaccinated the interpreters' children with *lympha* and Narabayashi Kensaburō with the *pokroven*. Kensaburō's vaccination was the only one that "took." It was a moment of personal and professional triumph for Narabayashi Sōken: he had worked with the Dutch for thirty years to try to bring cowpox vaccine to Japan, and it was he who had asked the Dutch to send the vaccine in the form of crusts or scabs.

Eleven days later Levyssohn wrote in the *Dagregister*: "The inoculation performed on the fourteenth of this month by Dr. Mohnike was—to the joy of the Japanese—successful with some Japanese children."[4] Mohnike later would write:

> In August 1849, thanks to the kindness of Dr. Bosch, Head of the Medical Service in the Netherlands Indies, I received a new quantity of vaccine, partly dry scabies, partly liquid lymph in tubes. Through this material vaccination was introduced to the thirty-five million people of Japan, even in the most northern part of the country thousands of children have been vaccinated.[5]

The fact that only one of the three vaccinations performed at Dejima was successful meant that the entire supply of cowpox vaccine in Japan was contained in the pocks on the arm of Narabayashi Kensaburō. It was imperative to reproduce the virus and increase the supply of vaccine as quickly as possible. This meant finding other children to vaccinate. Using the arm-to-arm method, and beginning with cowpox lymph taken from Kensaburō's arm, Mohnike spent the next three weeks vaccinating Nagasaki children. Then he focused on sending vaccine to other parts of Kyushu. On August 31, Mohnike asked Levyssohn to make the following recommendations to the Nagasaki authorities:

> For the purpose of speeding up the introduction of cowpox inoculation to the entire Japanese empire, already in its third generation of children inoculated by me from arm to arm, and because according to existing [Japanese] institutions I am not allowed to negotiate about this with the Nagasaki authorities myself, I request Your Honour to propose the following to the Governor of Nagasaki: That the Governor of Nagasaki send, via the agents and *chargé d'affaires* of the Lords of this large island who reside here [at Nagasaki], for one physician and several children who have not yet had smallpox from each district of Kyushu. This measure would not only give me the best opportunity to show physicians from other places how to perform the inoculation,

about the dangers and the progression of the vaccine pox, and all further matters concerning cowpox inoculation, but also how to transport viable lymph on the arms of children who are inoculated, which is the . . . surest way to move the inoculation material from one place to another.[6]

It was more prudent to move the children than to move the vaccine. Moving the *vaccinia* virus in the August heat and humidity of southwestern Japan would have risked losing the effectiveness of the vaccine. Mohnike's choice—to bring both physicians and children from other Kyushu domains to be vaccinated in Nagasaki—shows extreme caution and his awareness of the limits of his jurisdiction. Once children from other parts of Kyushu had been successfully vaccinated in Nagasaki, they were returned to their home domains to establish new sources of the vaccine.

Transporting children across domain lines—especially children infected with a visible pox disease—would surely have caused problems had the appropriate authorities not prepared the way beforehand. By gaining the approval of the Governor of Nagasaki, the shogun's deputy in Nagasaki and the highest-ranking local official, Mohnike had taken the necessary first step in the transmission of the vaccine virus from Nagasaki to other parts of Japan.

Levyssohn acted quickly. On the following day, he wrote to the Governor of Nagasaki emphasizing the benefits of vaccination and forwarding Mohnike's request:

> With the Dutch trade vessel currently here some cowpox material has been brought in and the Dutch physician at Deshima has used this material to inoculate some Japanese children. This inoculation was not only successful but is now already in its third generation. . . . In order to preserve this invention that is so beneficial to humanity and that has at last been successfully imported into Japan by the Dutch government, and in order to spread this invention quickly over the entire Japanese Empire, the undersigned Dutch Opperhoofd proposes to Your Honour: to have the agents of the lords of the island of Kyushu who live at Nagasaki bring here from every district a physician and some children who have not yet been affected or contaminated by the smallpox disease. Not only will this measure enable the Japanese physicians to become familiar with all aspects of inoculation, but also there is no safer way to transport the cowpox material from one place to another but on the arms of children who have been inoculated with viable vaccine.[7]

The speed and efficiency with which the diffusion of vaccination took place once it reached Nagasaki are truly remarkable. Many years of anticipation must have helped. Levyssohn, Mohnike, and their Japanese collaborators in Nagasaki—principally Dutch interpreters and *ranpō* physicians—initiated the dissemination of vaccine from Kyushu, but the national diffusion of vaccination was carried out by *ranpō* physicians who lived in Japan's many towns and villages.

THE KYUSHU DIFFUSION

Kyushu daimyo were already sympathetic to Western ideas, especially Western medical ideas with which they were well acquainted, and Mohnike's dissemination strategy worked well. It was not uncommon for *daimyō* to retain *ranpō* physicians on their medical staffs, and some *daimyō* had been engaged in the campaign to import the cowpox virus. Nabeshima Naomasa (1814–1871), Lord of Saga domain, is an excellent example. The Nabeshima family was one of Japan's highest-ranking *daimyō* families in terms of wealth and status, a powerful lineage that had supported Western learning for many years.[8] The Nabeshima belonged to a special land-holding category known as *kokushu,* which had special privileges and responsibilities, and the family had extensive holdings in Hizen Province.[9] The Nabeshima lords were responsible for the defense of Nagasaki, a responsibility they shared with the Gotō and Ōmura domain lords—also of Hizen Province—and with the Kuroda *daimyō* in neighboring Chikuzen Province.[10] Nabeshima Naomasa had become Lord of Saga domain in 1830, at sixteen years of age, when he inherited the family headship.[11] In 1849, he was a leading supporter of *rangaku* scholars, and he had several *ranpō* physicians—including Itō Genboku in Edo—on his medical staff.[12]

When Naomasa learned that cowpox vaccine had arrived in Nagasaki, he sent his personal physician, Ōishi Ryōei, to learn from Otto Mohnike how to perform vaccination. Ōishi Ryōei returned to Saga with Narabayashi Sōken's eldest son, Nagayoshi, who had been recently vaccinated in Nagasaki. On October 8, 1849, Ōishi Ryōei took lymph from a pock on Narabayashi Nagayoshi's arm and vaccinated Naomasa's eldest son and heir, Nabeshima Jun'ichirō.[13]

This simple tranmission of *V. vaccinae* from the arm of one child to the arm of another was not unlike the thousands of vaccinations that had been performed throughout the world during the previous half-century. Ōishi Ryōei used the same technique that Edward Jenner had used fifty years earlier when he took cowpox matter from the arm of Sarah Nelmes and implanted it in the arm of James Phipps. These two vaccinations have been memorialized in Japan and Britain, respectively, as events of marked historical significance— which indeed they were. But the similarity and significance of those two vaccinations end there.

The contexts were very different. In 1796, Jenner was conducting a new experiment to test a hypothesis—that inoculation with cowpox would prevent smallpox. In 1849, Jenner's hypothesis had been widely tested and verified. Nabeshima Naomasa knew that vaccination had been accepted throughout the world, and his decision to vaccinate his eldest son demonstrated both his knowledge and his conviction. Naomasa's decision also made a strong political statement. First, as one of Japan's greatest lords, he gave his stamp of approval to the imported practice of Jennerian vaccination. Second, by successfully vaccinating his own son and heir, he declared that vaccination was safe and the proper thing for a responsible parent to do. Third, by vaccinating his own son he gained the moral authority to order the vaccination of the children under his jurisdiction. Finally, the timing of his action was important. By acting shortly after the arrival of the vaccine, Naomasa gave invaluable support to the *ranpō* physicians who quickly needed to find other children to vaccinate in order to maintain a supply of live vaccine in Japan.

A large, handsome oil painting depicts the vaccination of Nabeshima Jun'ichirō at Saga Castle (Figure 6.1). The painting conveys both the concrete and the symbolic aspects of this important ceremony. It clearly illustrates the transmission of the vaccine: Naomasa stands behind his young son, who is seated at the center with his left arm and shoulder exposed. The young boy looks entirely serene as his mother looks on and Ōishi Ryōei prepares to prick his arm with a lancet. Narabayashi Nagayoshi is seated in the right foreground. His shoulder is also bare, and his left arm reveals a vaccination lesion from which Ryōei is about to take lymph to vaccinate the younger boy. There is no question about what is happening. The viewer observes the direct arm-to-arm transmission of *V. vaccinae* from donor to recipient and simultaneously witnesses the depiction of the traditional bond between lord and retainer in Tokugawa Japan: the retainer, Narabayashi Sōken, offers precious tribute—*V. vaccinae*—to his lord, Nabeshima Naomasa, to guarantee the life of his lord's son and heir.

The painting, of course, is commemorative. It was painted in 1927, long after the event it portrays, to memorialize the introduction of vaccination to

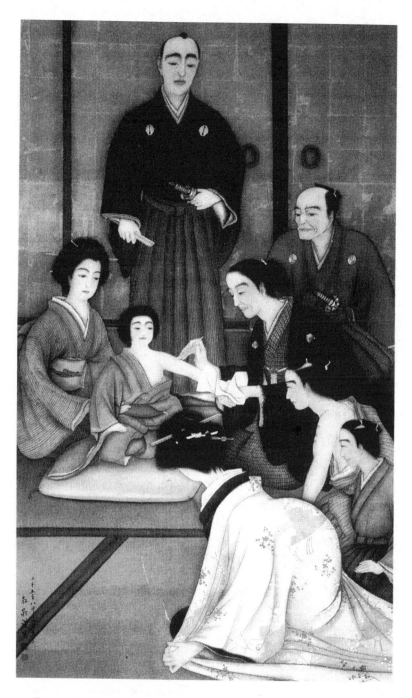

Figure 6.1. Vaccination at Saga Castle, 1849. Painting by Jinnouchi
Shōrei, 1927. Photograph courtesy of Saga Castle, Saga Prefectural
History Museum.

Japan, and to emphasize the critical role that Saga domain played in its diffusion.[14] It depicts quite effectively the close collaboration between *ranpō* physicians, *daimyō,* and other domain officials as they accomplished the successful dissemination of Jennerian vaccination.

In the subsequent weeks and months, similar, if less formal, ceremonies took place all over Japan as physicians first vaccinated their own children and then the children of local elites.[15] As in Europe, elites promoted the dissemination of both variolation and vaccination. What was unusual in Japan is that vaccination did not have the support of Japan's rulers, the Tokugawa *bakufu.* *Ranpō* physicians had organized both the importation of the vaccine and the diffusion of vaccination, and they did this without the involvement of their Tokugawa overlords. Rather, they marshaled the support of local and regional authorities who used their authority to order the vaccination of children under their jurisdiction. What is of particular interest is that Japan's vaccinators used the existing Tokugawa system of divided political authority—devised two and a half centuries earlier to forestall regional opposition movements—to launch a national movement from regional foci.

Among the *ranpō* physicians who responded to Mohnike's call to report to Nagasaki was Nagayo Shuntatsu, a physician from Ōmura domain, who had been interested in vaccination for thirty years. Having read a treatise about the cowpox method in the 1830s, he had tried to "create" cowpox by inoculating cows with smallpox.[16] When these attempts failed, he began to practice variolation instead. He opened a variolation retreat at Furutayama, in the mountains of Ōmura, where he inoculated children with smallpox virus. Shuntatsu, now sixty years old, participated in the Kyushu diffusion. When he learned that live cowpox vaccine had arrived on a Dutch ship, he went to Nagasaki to learn the cowpox method of inoculation. He then returned to Ōmura, converted his Furutayama facility into a vaccination clinic, and later initiated a revenue system that collected funds from domain villages to defray the costs of preserving and distributing viable cowpox vaccine.[17]

* * *

The Dutch considered the Kyushu diffusion a great success. In a letter to Levysshon dated November 11, 1849, Mohnike reports on how his strategy to involve the Kyushu *daimyō* and physicians in the dissemination of cowpox was progressing:

I thank Your Honour for your forceful co-operation in the introduction to the Japanese and the distribution among them of cowpox inoculation. This is a matter of the utmost importance for me as a human being and as a physician. I am pleased to inform Your Honour that at Nagasaki and in the other towns and districts of the island of Kyushu vaccination has taken root so well that we may hope that this wonderful invention will not only never be lost, but even that it will spread over the entire Japanese empire. At Nagasaki vaccine pocks already exist in their thirteenth generation—in nineteen children whom I have inoculated today—and the entire number of children inoculated by me from week to week since 14 August until now has reached 176. Apart from this, I have had Japanese physicians inoculate children in the areas outside Nagasaki. From the arms of children who were inoculated here, cowpox has already been transported to the provinces of Hizen and Shimabara. There the rulers have taken very wise measures to distribute the cowpox among all their subjects to keep it from disappearing again.[18]

Mohnike acknowledged the important role played by the regional *daimyō;* however, the real key to the success of the Kyushu diffusion was the involvement of Japan's *ranpō* physicians who had educated the *daimyō* about the benefits of vaccination well before the vaccine arrived in Nagasaki. Their knowledge and their connections to *ranpō* physicians in other parts of Japan would make it possible to extend the diffusion of vaccination well beyond Kyushu.

THE NATIONAL DIFFUSION

By the time Mohnike wrote to Levyssohn, the vaccine had already spread well beyond Kyushu. Map 6.1 shows the spatial diffusion of vaccine in 1849 from Nagasaki to other regions and towns in Japan. Within a few weeks vaccine had arrived in Japanese cities—Kyoto, Osaka, Fukui, and Edo—and these urban centers quickly became vaccine distributions centers for nearby towns and villages.

On October 22, Egawa Shirōhachi, a Chinese interpreter living in Nagasaki, sent cowpox crusts to Hino Teisai in Kyoto. He must have believed that it was safer to send crusts instead of lymph, and it was certainly simpler than sending a vaccinated child. Within twelve days the vaccine had arrived safely in Kyoto. Meanwhile, Kasahara Hakuō had received word in Fukui that cowpox vaccine had arrived in Nagasaki, and he left immediately for Kyushu. He

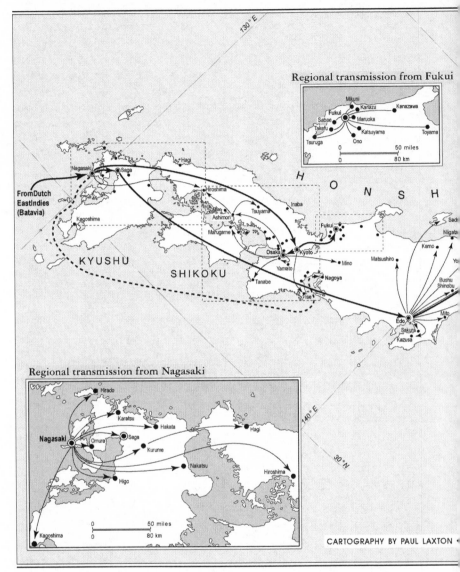

Map 6.1. National Transmission of Cowpox Vaccine from Nagasaki, 1849.

reached Kyoto in mid-November and stopped to visit his former teacher, Hino Teisai.[19] When Hakuō found out that Teisai had already received vaccine from Nagasaki, he stayed in Kyoto and helped him open a vaccination clinic. The Hakushin Jotōkan (Vaccine Inoculation Institute), Kyoto's first vaccination clinic, opened on November 30.[20] Meanwhile, Narabayashi

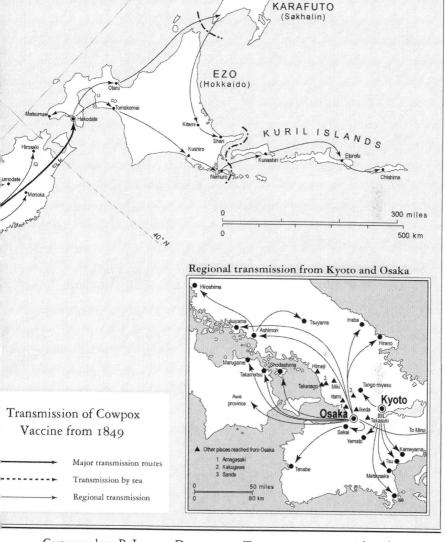

Transmission of Cowpox
Vaccine from 1849

———→ Major transmission routes

·–·–·–·▶ Transmission by sea

———→ Regional transmission

Regional transmission from Kyoto and Osaka

Cartographer, P. Laxton. Data source: *Tennentō no zero e no michi*, 36–39.

Eiken, Sōken's brother, now practicing and teaching medicine in Kyoto, had
also received vaccine from Nagasaki; and he too opened a Kyoto vaccination
clinic at his private medical school, Yūshindō.[21]

Ogata Kōan soon learned that there was cowpox vaccine in Kyoto, and on
December 15, he and two other Osaka physicians also went to visit Hino

Teisai. The three physicians stayed in Kyoto for several days to observe vaccinations at Teisai's clinic. A week later they returned to Osaka with live cowpox virus, and Ogata Kōan opened a vaccination clinic in Osaki at Tekijuku. When a good supply of vaccine had been secured through successive vaccinations in Kyoto and Osaka, the virus was divided further and shared with physicians in towns throughout the Kansai region.[22] The regional distribution of cowpox vaccine from Kyoto and Osaka to physicians in nearby towns can be seen in the right-hand corner of Map 6.1.[23]

Kasahara Hakuō stayed with Hino Teisai in Kyoto for two months, but as winter approached he prepared to return to Fukui. To optimize his chances of arriving in Fukui with live virus, he prepared carefully for the trip across the mountains. Hakuō summoned a family from Fukui—a father, mother, and two children—and hired a Kyoto family of four to accompany him part of the way. On December 30, he vaccinated the two Kyoto children and waited three days for the vaccination pocks to develop. He set out on his journey with a group of ten—the two families and an assistant. On January 5, a week after performing the Kyoto vaccinations in Kyoto, Hakuō took lymph from the now ripe pocks on the arms of the two Kyoto children and vaccinated the two Fukui children. He then sent the Kyoto family home. The remaining six members of the party continued on the next day, crossed the mountains in a winter snowstorm, and arrived in Fukui on January 8.

Kasahara Hakuō's detailed account of the Kyoto-Fukui transmission may appear compulsive; however, many who participated in the transmission of the vaccine kept records of where, when, and from whom they had received vaccine, and precisely what they had done with it. As noted earlier, good record keeping was essential to controlling the spread of smallpox everywhere, but in Japan during 1849, vaccination records were important for preventing the loss of viable vaccine. The Japanese were acutely aware of how difficult it had been to obtain cowpox virus, and that it would be no simple matter to acquire vaccine from abroad again. Consequently, they monitored the progress and whereabouts of the vaccine, and, without any official institution to require that they do so, they documented the successes and failures of vaccination. Many of these records have been preserved in local archives, because they document local initiative, collaboration across regional divisions, and the remarkable achievement that the Japanese associate with the introduction of vaccination to Japan. The careful records kept by those who conveyed the vaccine from place to place are what makes it possible today to reconstruct the networks that participated in the national diffusion of vaccination in Japan.

Kasahara Hakuō kept his account of the Kyoto-Fukui transmission in a personal diary entitled *Senkyō roku*, which covers the period from late October 1849 to 1853.[24] The diary begins with Hakuō's preparations for leaving Fukui to procure cowpox lymph. It explains how he and Hino Teisai set up the vaccination clinic in Kyoto, how they divided the vaccine virus with Ogata Kōan, and how he used the arm-to-arm method to convey vaccine from Kyoto to Fukui. Like his colleagues in Kyoto and Osaka, Kasahara Hakuō quickly opened a vaccination clinic in Fukui and began distributing cowpox vaccine to physicians in towns and villages along the coast of the Japan Sea. Map 6.1 shows the separate pattern of dissemination from Fukui.

THE EDO DIFFUSION

Meanwhile, *V. vaccinae* had already arrived in Edo. Nabeshima Naomasa took it himself when he went to Edo on his regularly scheduled journey to attend the shogun. Naomasa's responsibility for the defense of Nagasaki required that his attendance on the shogun fall between the eleventh and second months, when foreign ships were unlikely to come into the port.[25] Naomasa arrived in Edo on November 13 and took the vaccine to his Saga domain residence (*yashiki*) in Edo. The trajectory of direct transmission of the vaccine from Saga to Edo is shown in Map 6.1. Naomasa gave the vaccine to his physician-retainer, Itō Genboku, who shared the vaccine with other *ranpō* physicians in Edo. Ōtsuki Shunsai and Genboku were neighbors in Edo's Shitaya district, and Shunsai was probably among the first to receive the vaccine. They both began vaccinating children in their homes. Ōtsuki Shunsai, now a physician-retainer for Sendai domain, also vaccinated officials' children in the Sendai domain *yashiki*.[26]

Itō Genboku vaccinated Naomasa's daughter, Nabeshima Mitsuhime, at the Saga *yashiki* in Edo on December 25, 1849. Genboku made twelve small wounds—two rows of three on each arm.[27] Multiple vaccination sites on both arms became the standard procedure, a technique that may have differed from that taught by Otto Mohnike. As in the case of the vaccination at Saga Castle, witnesses were present at the vaccination ceremony, and their names were recorded for posterity. Ōishi Ryōei, who had vaccinated Naomasa's son in Saga, was in attendance, as were at least three other *ranpō* physicians.[28] Ryōei may have been present to see that the vaccination was done properly. The others may have been there to learn how to perform the technique.

The vaccination of Mitsuhime at Saga domain's official residence in Edo emphasizes the dominant role of Saga in the *national* diffusion of vaccination. When Nabeshima Naomasa took V. *vaccinae* to Edo, he was taking it to the very center of *bakufu*-controlled territory. Naomasa had authorized the vaccinations of his son in Saga and his daughter in Edo. Despite the fact that the practice of Western medicine had been banned in all *bakufu* territories, he did not seek permission nor did he experience any interference from the Edo government.

Naomasa was not the only domain lord to vaccinate children in their Edo residences. Hotta Masayoshi of Sakura domain used his Edo *yashiki* as a vaccine distribution center for the children of his domain. His official biography, published in 1922, states that Hotta Masayoshi, like Nabeshima Naomasa, had his own children vaccinated first. When he observed that they came to no harm, he ordered a general vaccination of the children of Sakura domain, and he sent children to Edo to be vaccinated and to bring vaccine back to Sakura. Watanabe Yaichibei, Masayoshi's deputy at that time, wrote in January 1850: "we were again hearing about cowpox and I sent my own young daughters to Edo to be vaccinated; . . . somewhat later vaccination laws were announced stating that all the people in the domain—rich and poor alike—were to be vaccinated."[29]

Watanabe issued instructions urging local officials throughout the domain to proceed with vaccination. But this was not so easily accomplished:

> People everywhere were afraid of this danger and hesitated, and anxious that Masayoshi's concern for his people should come to naught, the district officials gave strict orders to the village officials that they must not stop [vaccinating]. [Parents] tearfully brought out their beloved children to receive the vaccine.[30]

The benefits of vaccination were not immediately clear, and the *daimyō* who had ordered the vaccination of the children under their jurisdiction had to wait until the next smallpox epidemic to demonstrate that vaccination really did prevent smallpox. According to Watanabe, only when smallpox again struck a town or village could everyone observe that "the children who had been vaccinated did not get the infection, while those who had not been vaccinated continued, one after the other, to become infected. When the effectiveness of vaccination was generally understood, there was a scramble to be first in line—with people begging to be vaccinated."[31]

Collaboration between the physicians of domains in different parts of Japan made it possible for vaccinations to be performed in Edo in domain *yashiki* without the involvement of the *bakufu*. The vaccine brought by Nabeshima Naomasa of Saga domain was shared with other *daimyō* and domain officials, which made it possible for the virus to proceed outward from the capital to domains throughout northeastern Japan.

Official domain residences were not the only places in Edo where vaccinations could be performed. Both Itō Genboku and Ōtsuki Shunsai gave vaccine to other Edo physicians, who then vaccinated their private patients. The most enthusiastic of these physicians was Kuwata Ryūsai, the adopted son of Kuwata Genshin. Both father and son had been performing variolation in Edo's Fukagawa district for many years, but when Genboku gave Kuwata Ryūsai cowpox vaccine, reportedly on January 1, 1850, Ryūsai immediately switched to vaccination. He quickly would become Edo's most creative vaccination advocate.

The ease with which Japanese *ranpō* physicians were able to switch from variolation to vaccination suggests a significant difference from the way vaccination was received in the West, where variolators and vaccinators were fierce competitors. Among *ranpō* physicians who used it, variolation was always regarded as inferior to vaccination. Thus, as soon as cowpox vaccine became available, vaccination immediately became the method of choice.

* * *

Within six months of the arrival of the vaccine—by the end of 1849 (Ka'ei 2)—Japanese medical historians claim that vaccination had been introduced to all the provinces of Japan.[32] This claim is difficult to prove; however, it is clear that cowpox vaccine did reach all major regions of Japan within this short period. The national network of *ranpō* physicians and their many collaborators had acted quickly and effectively.

Table 6.1 is a chronology of important benchmarks in the transmission of cowpox vaccine in Japan. It documents the timing of the distribution of the vaccine from Nagasaki and identifies the key individuals and places that served as the links in the transmission. It complements the spatial transmission represented in Map 6.1. The chronology compiles information from both

TABLE 6.1

A chronology of the transmission of vaccination, 1849–1850

1849	Ka'ei 2	Events
8.11	6.23	Vaccine arrives at Nagasaki.[a]
8.14	6.26	Otto Mohnike, Dejima physician, vaccinates three Japanese children at the home of Nagasaki physician Narabayashi Sōken.[b]
8.25	7.8	Opperhoofd Joseph Henrij Levyssohn reports the success of vaccination with "some" Japanese children.[c]
8.31	7.14	Mohnike asks Levyssohn to ask the Governor of Nagasaki to bring children from Kyushu domains to be vaccinated.
9.1	7.15	Levyssohn writes to the Governor of Nagasaki.[d]
9.24	8.8	Vaccination arrives in Saga domain, Hizen Province.[e]
10.8	8.22	Oishi Ryōei uses cowpox matter from the arm of Narabayashi Naga-yoshi, to vaccinate the son of Nabeshima Naomasa, Lord of Saga domain, Nabeshima Jun'ichirō, at Saga Castle.[f]
10.22	9.6	Egawa Shirōhachi, a Chinese interpreter in Nagasaki, sends vaccine to Hino Teisai in Kyoto.[g]
11.3	9.19	Hino Teisai receives the vaccine in Kyoto;[h] Kasahara Hakuō leaves Fukui for Nagasaki.[i]
11.5	9.21	Miyake Gonsai vaccinates children in Hiroshima.[j]
11.6	9.22	Nabeshima Naomasa leaves Saga for Edo with cowpox vaccine.[k]
11.11	9.27	Mohnike reports to Levyssohn that he has performed 176 successful vaccinations in Nagasaki.[l]
11.13	9.29	Nabeshima Naomasa arrives in Edo.[m]
11.19	10.5	Kasahara Hakuō joins Hino Teisai in Kyoto.[n] Levyssohn writes reports to the Governor-General at Batavia on the progress of vaccination in Japan.[o]
11.30	10.16	Hino Teisai and Kasahara Hakuō opened Kyoto's first vaccination clinic, the Hakushin Jotōkan, with the vaccination of six children; this public event was attended by public officials and local dignitaries.[p]
11.	10.	Narabayashi Eiken opens a vaccination clinic at Yūshindō in Kyoto.[q]
12.15	11.1	Ogata Kōan and two other physicians take children from Osaka to Hino Teisai in Kyoto to be vaccinated. They stay for several days to be certain the vaccinations took and then return to Kyoto.[r]
12.21	11.7	Ogata Kōan holds a formal ceremony to open a vaccination clinic at Tekijuku in Osaka.[s]
12.25	11.11	Itō Genboku vaccinates Nabeshima Naomasa's daughter, Mitsuhime, at the Saga domain *yashiki* in Edo.[t]
12.30	11.16	Kasahara Hakuō vaccinates two Kyoto children to assist with the transmission of vaccine to Fukui.[u]
1850	**Ka'ei 2**	
1.1	11.18	Itō Genboku gives the vaccine to Kuwata Ryūsai.[v]
1.2	11.19	Kasahara Hakuō leaves Kyoto for Fukui with two Kyoto children and two Fukui children.[w]

1.5	11.22	Kasahara Hakuō vaccinates two Fukui children and sends the Kyoto children home[x]
1.8	11.25	Kasahara Hakuō introduces vaccination to Fukui and the Japan Sea coastal region.[y]
1.13	12.	Itō Keisuke introduces vaccination in Nagoya with vaccine brought from Nagasaki by Shibata Hōan.[z]
	12.	Hotta Masayoshi sends children to Edo be vaccinated and to bring vaccine to Sakura (Chiba Prefecture) domain.[aa]

a. NFJ 1618: n.p. *Dagregister*, entry for August 14, 1849.
b. *Tennentō*, 106, gives Ka'ei 2.7.17 (September 3, 1849) as the date of these vaccinations.
c. NFJ 1632/36: Mohnike to Levyssohn, August 31, 1849.
d. NFJ 1649/29: Levysshon to the Governor of Nagasaki, September 1, 1849.
e. *Tennentō*, 38-39.
f. Ibid., 106; Soekawa, 23.
g. Soekawa, 23.
h. *Tennentō*, 106.
i. Kasahara Hakuō, *Senkyō roku*, 1.
j. *Tennentō*, 106.
k. Ibid., 39.
l. NFJ 1632/36: Mohnike to Levyssohn, November 11, 1849.
m. *Tennentō*, 39.
n. Ibid., 106. Kasahara, 2.
o. NFJ 1632/36: Mohnike to Levyssohn, November 11, 1849.
p. Kasahara, 3; *Tennentō*, 38, 106; Ishida Sumio, *Ogata Kōan no rangaku (Ogata Kōan and Dutch Studies)* (Kyoto: Shibunkaku Shuppan, 1992), 17.
q. *Tennentō*, 38.
r. Kasahara, 5.
s. Ibid., 6. *Tennentō*, 106.
t. Ibid., 39, 106.
u. Kasahara, 7.
v. *Yōgaku shi jiten*, 240.
w. Kasahara, 9.
x. Ibid.
y. Ibid., 9; *Tennentō*, 106.
z. Ibid., 39.
aa. Ogawa Teizō, 83.

NOTE: Conversion of calendar dates is based on Uchida Masao, compiler, *Nihon rekijitsu genten* (Tokyo: Yūzankaku, 1975-1981).

Dutch and Japanese sources, which are dated according to different calendar systems; therefore, dates, when known, are given in both Western and Japanese calendars.[33] This chronology makes it abundantly clear that once cowpox vaccine was exported from Nagasaki to other places in Japan, the diffusion of vaccination was an entirely Japanese affair.

The large discrepancy between dates in the Western (Gregorian) and Japanese calendars in 1849 complicates the transmission story and requires explanation.[34] All months in the old Japanese solar-lunar calendar had either twenty-nine or thirty days. Every three to four years the official lunar calendar had to be adjusted to bring it into accord with the solar calendar—that is, with the occurrences of the winter and summer solstices and the cycle of the four seasons. This adjustment was made by adding, or "intercalating," a thirteenth

month of thirty days every three to four years. Ka'ei 2 (1849) was an inter-
calary, thirteen-month year: an extra fourth month was intercalated between
the fourth and fifth month. Hence, during the months when cowpox virus was
being hand-carried from place to place (between the sixth month and the end
of the year), the discrepancy between dates in the Western and Japanese calendars was almost two months. For example, when the vaccine arrived in Nagasaki, the date was recorded in the Dutch records as August 14, 1849 (1849,
eighth month, fourteenth day); that same date in the Japanese calendar was
Ka'ei 2.6.26 (second year, sixth month, twenty-sixth day of the Ka'ei era).

Western and Japanese dates for a particular event do not always agree; in
fact, different Japanese records sometimes disagree about the date a particular
event took place. It must be remembered that many people were recording
what was happening in many different localities, and small discrepancies are
to be expected.

The discrepancy in recorded dates can influence one's interpretation of
what occurred. A casual reading of the Japanese calendar dates would suggest that dissemination of the vaccine took place in the summer and early
autumn, the hottest months of the year in Japan when the heat-sensitive
cowpox virus would have had the greatest difficulty surviving. The Western
calendar dates, however, confirm that the transmission of cowpox vaccine in
Japan was accomplished in the autumn and early winter, a far more propitious time to transport live vaccine virus. The calendar conversion is well
worthwhile, because the meticulous attention to detail in the Japanese accounts provide us with a remarkably clear picture of the timing and the trajectory of the transmission of the cowpox virus in Japan in 1849.

Was there a need to keep such detailed accounts? The answer is closely related to the nature of the logistical task the vaccinators faced. As long as the
arm-to-arm method was the only reliable way to vaccinate children, recently
vaccinated children were the sole source of vaccine. These children were required to return to vaccination clinics to be checked; if their vaccinations had
"taken," they were required to donate fresh vaccine so that others could be vaccinated.[35] A successful vaccination clinic had to monitor the comings and go-
ings of potential donors and recipients very closely, because the optimum time
to take lymph from a vaccination pock was a very narrow window, around the
eighth day after vaccination. Obviously, accurate records were essential for the
effective management of vaccination clinics, and Japan's excellent vaccination
records demonstrate just how well the vaccinators understood their task.

The rapid diffusion of vaccination was dramatic and highly visible, and before long everyone could observe its benefits. The long prohibition against contact with foreigners made the Dutch a more formidable intellectual presence than might otherwise have been the case. Had vaccination come to Japan through normal commercial or diplomatic intercourse with China half a century earlier, its impact would probably have been quite different. With the strong support for Chinese-style medicine perpetrated by the official medical establishment in Edo, vaccination might well have been viewed as a Chinese innovation. The enormous difficulties that had to be overcome to obtain *V. vaccinae* from the Dutch, on the other hand, meant that the benefits of vaccination were attributed to the heroic efforts of *ranpō* physicians and the superiority of Western medicine. The introduction of vaccination by the Dutch glorified both Western medicine and those who espoused it.

EDUCATING PHYSICIANS

The fate of vaccination could not rely indefinitely on a loosely constructed network of colleagues, patrons, and friends, however enthusiastic they might be. The transmission of *V. vaccinae* was only the initial step in confronting smallpox. Before vaccination could immunize the large number of young children who were susceptible to the disease, the situation demanded an exponential increase in the number of vaccinators. When the vaccine became available, it was essential to transmit reliable and practical information about vaccination to medical personnel and to the public. While word-of-mouth transmission was clearly important, the publication of books about vaccination played a major role.

When the vaccine virus arrived in the summer of 1849, there was virtually no published information on the subject of vaccination. Yet within six months, many informative and useful books on vaccination were in print. The almost instantaneous appearance of books of instruction and commentary about vaccination is as remarkable as the speed with which the cowpox vaccine penetrated the Japanese Islands. How was this accomplished so quickly?

The rapid publication of books on vaccination provides the most convincing evidence of an active network of physicians whose knowledge of vaccination spanned several decades. Several of these books were much earlier translations of Western writings on vaccination that had been hand-copied and circulated among a small group of medical scholars as unpublished manuscripts. As cow-pox vaccine was traveling between Japan's villages and towns, these unpub-lished works were being dusted off and published. They were revised, edited, and published with new prefaces, forewords, afterwords, appendices, and com-mentary. Many were given new titles, a common practice that greatly compli-cates the task of those who now try to establish a book's provenance.

One of the earliest translations, published in 1849, was Baba Sajūrō's "Tonka hiketsu," the translation of the Russian vaccination tract that he had completed in 1820 (see Chapter 3). An Edo physician named Toshimitsu Sen'an revised and published this early translation as *Roshia gyūtō zensho* (*A Russian Book on Cowpox*) in 1850.[36] Sen'an explains in his preface to the book that he had bought a copy of "Tonka hiketsu" in Nagasaki twenty years earlier and had kept it in his possession since that time.[37] The fact that Toshimitsu Sen'an was able to buy a copy of Baba Sajūrō's treatise within a few years of the latter's death in 1822 suggests that Sajūrō's translation of the Russian tract had been copied and was circulating privately. Furthermore, the fact that an Edo physician bought Sajūrō's book in the late 1820s suggests that the impor-tance of his treatise was already recognized and appreciated well beyond the small circle of official interpreters to which Baba Sajūrō belonged.

According to the custom of the time, Toshimitsu Sen'an wrote his preface in classical Chinese. His other contributions to this small volume, however—a foreword and an afterword—are written in a colloquial style that was easy to read. Editors and copiers commonly made whatever changes they wished without acknowledging them, so it is unlikely that Toshimitsu Sen'an's ver-sion of "Tonka hiketsu" is an exact replica of Baba Sajūrō's original translation. Fortunately, however, Sen'an retained Sajūrō's original preface to the transla-tion in which the young interpreter relates how he had first learned about vac-cination in Nagasaki from his teacher, Hendrik Doeff, in the early 1800s; how in 1813 he obtained a copy of the Russian vaccination tract while serving as a government interpreter in Ezo; how in 1818 an English Captain had offered him cowpox lymph, lancets, and an instruction book (which he had to refuse); and why he decided to finish his translation of the Russian tract in 1820.

Sajūrō's straightforward account of the sequence of events that compelled him to finish his translation of the Russian book documents not only his own tenacity and his belief that what he had learned should not be lost, but also the efforts of Europeans who, for four decades, had tried to introduce Jennerian vaccination to Japan. By publishing Baba Sajūrō's story immediately after the arrival of the vaccine in 1849, Toshimitsu Sen'an was also exposing the fact that information about the benefits of vaccination had been available in Japan since the beginning of the century, and that no one had found a way to act upon this knowledge.[38]

Another Japanese translation to be published in 1849 also has an interesting history. This was based on the Dutch translation of the German book first published in Europe at the beginning of the nineteenth century: H. J. Goldschmidt's *Algemeene beschouwing van de geschiedenis der koepokken* . . . , published in Amsterdam in 1802.[39] As mentioned earlier, a copy of Goldschmidt's book had been sent from Batavia to Jan Cock Blomhoff in 1821, the book that the authorities at Batavia asked him to return more than once. Possibly he failed to do so; alternatively, another copy could have been brought or sent to Japan later. The translator of Goldschmidt's book was Arima Setsuzō (1817–1847), a student of Ogata Kōan who learned to read Dutch at Tekijuku. Since Tekijuku was not established until 1838, Arima Setsuzō most likely worked on this translation in the 1840s when Kōan's best students were working on Dutch medical translations. Arima Setsuzō called his translation *Gyūtō shinsho* (*A New Book About Cowpox*). He died in 1847, at age thirty, and his translation was published posthumously in 1850 after the vaccine arrived. Another student of Ogata Kōan, Hirose Genkyō (1821–1870), published a revised edition of Itō Keisuke's translation of Alexander Pearson's vaccination tract in 1850.[40] An illustration depicting the arm-to-arm method of vaccination, shown in Figure 6.2, is from this edition.

Many Japanese translations of Western writings on vaccination were never published. These included translations by prominent *ranpō* physicians such as Satō Taizen and Itō Genboku, who were actively involved in the dissemination of vaccination in 1849. These unpublished translations had served their purpose: they had educated and convinced their translators that vaccination was the best way of preventing smallpox, so when the vaccine did arrive, they spent their time promoting the technique. As Jenner had emphasized, vaccination was a simple procedure, anyone could be taught to vaccinate. There really was no need to publish old translations of Western or Chinese texts. Japan's vaccinators could write their own books based on their own experiences.

New Japanese books on vaccination were published almost simultaneously with the old translations. The first and most influential was Narabayashi Sōken's *Gyūtō shokō* (*Thoughts About Cowpox*), published in Nagasaki in 1849. As one of the earliest promoters of Jennerian vaccination, and as the father of

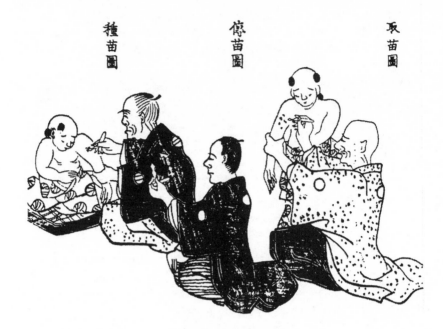

Figure 6.2. Depicting the Arm-to-Arm Method of Vaccination. Source: Hirose Genkyō, *Shintei gyūtō kihō*, 1850.

the first child in Japan to be successfully vaccinated, Narabayashi Sōken wrote persuasively. *Gyūtō shokō* is a twenty-four page, personal testimonial to the safety and effectiveness of vaccination. It tells how the cowpox virus was brought to Nagasaki, gives detailed instructions on how to perform vaccination, and includes an illustration showing a child with clearly marked vaccination sites on his arms. The drawing in Figure 6.3 shows a specially designed lancet with a slit at the point to hold the cowpox lymph. Sōken emphasized that these instructions were based on the teachings of the Dutch physician Otto Mohnike, thus clearly identifying vaccination with its Western origins, with the Dutch, and with the *rangaku* and *ranpō* communities in Japan.[41]

Kasahara Hakuō also wrote a manual about vaccination, *Gyūtō mondō,* and with financial assistance from a local Fukui merchant, he had it published by the Kyoto printing firm Kyūkōdō in 1850. Hakuō produced additional short notes and treatises about vaccination, which were not published at the time. These include his diary describing his journey from Kyoto to Fukui, and "Instructions on Vaccination" dated 1859. The latter was written for

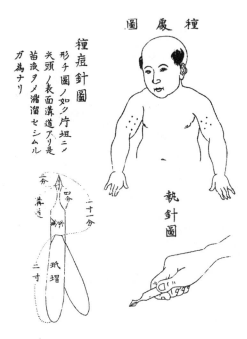

Figure 6.3. Depicting the Technique of Vaccination. Source: Narabayashi Sōken, *Gyūtō shutō*, 3.

local physicians to instruct them in the technique of vaccination and the sequential stages in the development of the characteristic pock. It was handcopied and distributed with samples of cowpox vaccine to physicians who practiced in villages along the Japan Sea.

Kuwata Ryūsai in Edo published at least two books on vaccination in 1849. He edited a one-volume version of *Intō shinpō zensho*, a book originally published in China and already translated by the *kanpō* physician Koyama Shisei. He called his abridged edition *Intō yō ryakkai* (*A Short Commentary on Vaccination*), a title very similar to the original Chinese. His intention was to make the information in the original Chinese text more accessible to Japanese physicians. Ryūsai did not share Koyama Shisei's antipathy toward Westerners. As a pediatrician and an experienced practitioner of variolation, Ryūsai had credentials in both *kanpō* and *ranpō* medicine. He was concerned not about where the vaccine had come from, but about how to prevent children from getting smallpox. Ryūsai may have finished editing *Intō yō ryakkai* before the vaccine arrived in Nagasaki. Later that same year he published *Gyūtō hatsumō* (*Overcoming Ignorance About Smallpox*), his own book on vaccination.

Gyūtō hatsumō departed from the established format for Japanese medical treatises. It opens with a table of simple statistics designed to prove that vaccination was a more effective way to prevent smallpox than variolation, and far better than waiting for smallpox to strike naturally. While the intended audience for this book may have been unconvinced physicians, it was written in language that would allow any reader to become informed. The book includes an appendix with a list of related works on vaccination, which identify the authors of unpublished manuscripts as well as published books by his medical colleagues. *Gyūtō hatsumō* was a scholarly analysis of what Ryūsai had learned about vaccination from the works of others, as well as a vaccination tract designed to publicize and promote vaccination in Japan.

The books published in the wake of the vaccine's arrival served to enlarge and extend the network of physicians and others who participated in the diffusion of vaccination. Merchants, publishers, and booksellers, as well as physicians, became involved in the process. These new books on vaccination often gave the names of vaccinating physicians in various locations, lists of titles and authors of additional books on vaccination, and even the names and locations of bookstores where these books could be bought.

CONVINCING THE PUBLIC

Informing the general public required a different sort of approach. If parents were to bring their children to physicians to be vaccinated, they needed not only to know about the promise of vaccination, but also to believe that it would not harm their children. Feudal lords may have been able to order their subjects to be vaccinated, but broad popular support for vaccination, especially in the cities, was required if there were to be enough children vaccinated to sustain and expand the vaccine supply. Many years would pass before it would be possible to create a stable supply of vaccine that did not depend on vaccinated children. But how to explain the benefits of vaccination to a populace that, for the most part, was not familiar with any form of inoculation? As in the case of Jenner's early experiments, parents had to be taught to replace fear with trust. Fear was a given: no one needed to be taught to fear smallpox. Trust had to be won.

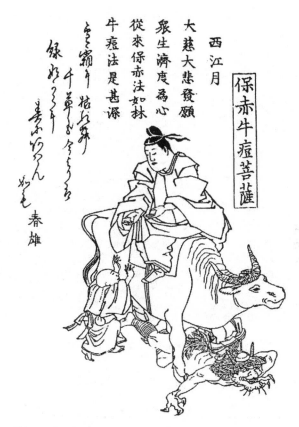

西江月
大慈大悲發願
眾生濟度為心
從來保赤法如林
牛痘法是甚諱

保赤牛痘菩薩

Figure 6.4. Bodhisattva Rescuing a Child from the
Smallpox Demon. Source: Frontispiece in Kuwata
Ryūsai, *Intō yō ryakkai*, 1849.

Kuwata Ryūsai may have been the most creative of the vaccinators in his
efforts to win the support of the public, perhaps because he was a pediatrician who regularly dealt with the hopes and fears of parents and children.
Also, as a pediatrician and smallpox specialist, he was not new to the practice
of inoculation. He had known about vaccination for most of his adult life,
and with his adoptive father he had been variolating children with smallpox
virus for many years. For Kuwata Ryūsai, replacing smallpox virus with
cowpox virus was a rather small step. He included familiar images in his
books, such as that of the Boddhisattva rescuing a child from the smallpox
demon, in Figure 6.4, to allay fears of a new and foreign technology.[42]

In early 1850, Kuwata Ryūsai commissioned and published an illustrated

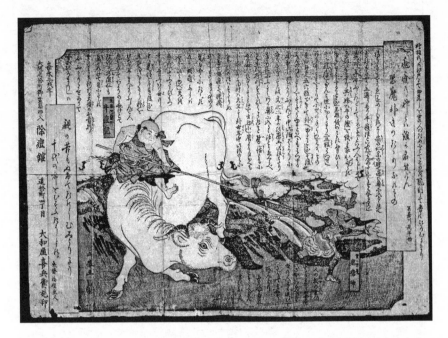

Figure 6.5. The Cowpox Child. Image courtesy of Kawaguchi Koichi and the Koga City Museum of History.

flyer with a simple message. This illustration, Figure 6.5, is an appealing, multicolored woodblock print showing a white cow grazing in a field. Sitting on the cow's back is a little boy who is poking a long stick at a small, dark smallpox demon that is trying to run away in fright. An inscription written in simple Japanese script (*katakana* and a few *kanji*) gives a short history of smallpox and vaccination and makes the following claims: formerly people thought that smallpox was caused by a deity, but this is not true. Smallpox is a disease, a disease that can now be prevented. Dr. Etoienneru [Edward Jenner] has discovered a new method, *gyūtō shutō* (cowpox inoculation) to prevent smallpox. This new method is better and safer than *jintō shutō* (smallpox inoculation), an older method that uses human pox.

The inscription explains that the cowpox virus arrived in China during the Bunsei Period (1818–1829) [this assertion is incorrect] and in Japan in Ka'ei 2 (1849). It then tells the story of Mitsuhime, the daughter of Nabeshima Naomasa, Lord of Saga, who had been recently inoculated with cowpox vaccine in Edo [by Itō Genboku]. Ryūsai concludes his story with a reassuring statement to parents: they could now find relief from their great anxiety about smallpox—so often fatal—by having their young children vaccinated before they were exposed to smallpox.

Kuwata Ryūsai's first cowpox print was dated Ka'ei 3.1, which would place it in circulation in Edo sometime between mid-February and mid-March 1850. Soekawa Masao believed that the early date on this print suggests that Kuwata Ryūsai's strong faith in vaccination may not have been based on personal experience. He did not, after all, receive vaccine from Itō Genboku until early January 1850.[43] However, he would have heard the early reports about successful vaccinations and he would have known the outcome of Nabeshima Mitsuhime's vaccination on December 25. By mid-February he would have had an opportunity to vaccinate many children and to have received encouraging reports from other sources as well.

Kuwata Ryūsai produced and distributed many thousands of his woodblock print during the early years of vaccination. The young boy riding the cow became known as the Cowpox Child, and Ryūsai's propaganda bills were called Cowpox Child prints by the people of Edo. Other physicians who wished to attract children to their clinics to be vaccinated were quick to follow Ryūsai's example. Ogata Kōan's vaccination clinic in Osaka distributed a print (fig. 6.5) almost identical to Ryūsai's later in 1850, and Kōan's inscription is very similar to Ryūsai's. Arguing against rumors stating that cowpox vaccination was not only ineffective but harmful—indicating that there was opposition—Kōan urged parents to bring their children to the clinic to be vaccinated. Interestingly, Kōan's print corrected Ryūsai's mistake about when the cowpox virus had first reached China, but he added a mistake of his own, claiming that Jenner had discovered the cowpox method in the Netherlands.[44] Cowpox prints with similar themes were soon being circulated by other Japanese physicians.[45] The rapid production of similar prints in Japan's cities shows that the connections between physicians, which had been activated to distribute the cowpox vaccine, continued to function so that children would be brought into their clinics to be vaccinated. These prints were an essential part of the effort to introduce vaccination to Japan, because maintaining a viable vaccine supply depended upon having children to vaccinate.

* * *

In stark contrast to the active involvement of several high-ranking domain lords, the *bakufu* appears to have ignored vaccination entirely. How to explain

such a peculiar reaction? Ignorance must be at least part of the answer. Vaccination was a widely acclaimed medical technique that could prevent smallpox
—a disease that could and did kill children of both the Tokugawa and imperial
families. But which of the shogun's advisors was going to enlighten him about
this? Hotta Masayoshi of Sakura and Matsudaira Shungaku of Fukui, two of
the most ardent supporters of vaccination, *were* advisors to the shogun. However, they chose to exercise their authority as *daimyō,* to order vaccinations in
their own domains and in their Edo *yashiki*—under the very noses of *bakufu*
officials. Neither influential *daimyō* nor well-placed *ranpō* physicians in Edo
sought *bakufu* support for vaccination after the vaccine had arrived.

The *daimyō* and others who privately advocated vaccination may have
thought it inadvisable to challenge the leadership of the Igakkan, the Tokugawa Medical College in Edo. The edict of April 7, 1849 (Ka'ei 2.3.15), pro-
hibiting the practice of Western medicine in Tokugawa territories, had been
issued shortly before the vaccine arrived. If questioned, one could always point
out that Western-style vaccination was, in fact, a surgical technique, and
Western surgery had been specifically excluded from the ban.[46] Even so, the
severity of recent and not-so-recent purges of important *rangaku* scholars and
ranpō physicians would have urged great caution. A second reason for avoid-
ing *bakufu* involvement was the precedent of Ogata Shunsaku, who had tried
unsuccessfully to promote variolation in *bakufu*-controlled territories in the
1790s. It may have seemed wise to avoid the risk of such an outcome in the
case of vaccination.

Another explanation comes to mind. The government's lack of involvement may not have been opposition to vaccination but tacit approval. Edo,
Kyoto, Osaka, and Nagasaki, the major centers of distribution for the vaccine,
were under the direct control of the *bakufu.* Any ban against Western medical
practices would have applied to each of those cities. Yet no official of the Edo
government made any effort to stop the transmission of V. *vaccinae* or the practice of vaccination in those cities. All things considered, the discreet, private,
semi-clandestine manner in which the vaccine was conveyed from place to
place may have been standard practice for trying out new ideas. Had problems
developed, no blame would fall on the *bakufu,* and those responsible could be
punished; if the ideas proved successful, the *bakufu* could think about adopting them.

A contemporary observation in 1851 by the Dutch physician Otto
Mohnike offers additional food for thought:

The central government at Edo is fully aware of the great importance of vaccination and secretly encourages its introduction but there still exists no official . . . policy for this. The government of Japan considers vaccination a foreign institution entering the country and therefore at odds with the policy of isolation. In spite of these circumstances the daimyo, who govern the entire empire apart from the largest cities and some towns and villages, have effectively taken measures for spreading vaccination among their subjects, without interference from the central government at Edo. The lords of Nagato, Echizen, Mito, Kaga, Sendai and others on Nippon, together with those of Satsuma, Hizen, Chikuzen, Ōmura, Shimabara, Higo, Takiwo [sic], etc. have issued strict orders that all children are to be vaccinated. To execute this they have appointed physicians in all districts and subdistricts who vaccinate at set times and without charge. So there is reason to believe that vaccine in Japan will not be lost. Some people believe that the Japanese government considers vaccination undesirable because it could lead to over-population, but I do not agree. The reason is that it conflicts with the old rule of isolation from foreign influences.[47]

Mohnike may well have been correct, although he seems not to have considered that had the Japanese government wished to do so, it could have imported vaccine from China many decades earlier. It should be remembered, however, that it was the Qing (Manchu) government that had fostered variolation and Qing physicians who had written the books promoting vaccination. In the eyes of the Japanese, the Qing government was not a Chinese government but a Manchu government, and the Japanese government regarded the Manchus as foreign barbarians.

Whatever the reasons may have been, the *bakufu*'s failure to engage in the introduction of vaccination to Japan may have been a blessing in disguise. Official oversight would have required rules, regulations, surveillance, and efforts to control the transmission of vaccine that would have been counterproductive. The network of knowledgeable physicians who had made it their business to learn all there was to know about vaccination was far more qualified to manage the transmission of *V. vaccinae* than a government that had remained aloof from the matter.

SEVEN

Engaging the Center

In the 1850s, the Western powers closed in from all sides with increasing demands for the shogun to negotiate commercial treaties and open Japan's ports to foreign trade. Commodore Matthew C. Perry of the United States Navy, who entered Uraga Bay with a fleet of American gunships to press the point in 1853, was the first to succeed. As factions for and against negotiating with the Western nations gained and lost favor, top officials in the Tokugawa *bakufu* changed rapidly. After a year the *bakufu* acquiesced to Perry's demands, and trade negotiations between the parties began. It was painfully obvious that the Edo government needed the expertise of persons knowledgeable about the West, particularly those who could read Western languages, to negotiate with the foreigners. Those most qualified were the *tenmonkata*, the government's official translators of Western books, most of whom were physicians. The demands on the *bakufu* after 1854 created unusual opportunities for these men to engage, for the first time, in activities that were unrelated to medicine. Physicians who had attempted to advise the *bakufu* on political matters had often been severely punished. This new engagement in political affairs gave physicians who wished to promote vaccination an opportunity to push their vaccination agenda forward.

Following the importation of the cowpox vaccine in 1849, the strategy of the Edo vaccinators for almost a decade had been to demonstrate that vaccination worked, that inoculation with cowpox vaccine really did prevent smallpox, and that vaccination was not harmful. They waited for a positive sign to seek the approval of the *bakufu*. That moment came in 1857 with two almost simultaneous developments: the deaths of the two most powerful opponents of Western medicine, Taki Motokata and Tsujimoto Shōan at the Igakkan, the Tokugawa medical school in Edo;[1] and the outbreak of a severe smallpox epidemic in Ezo and the domains of northeastern Honshu.

The Taki family had occupied the top posts at the Igakkan since 1765, when Shogun Tokugawa Ieharu made the Igakkan the Tokugawa *bakufu*'s official school of Chinese-style medicine. The Taki family was adamantly opposed to Western-style medicine, and was largely responsible for the escalating prohibitions against its practice in the 1840s. Taki Motokata and Tsujimoto Shōan had administered the Igakkan at that time, and their deaths in the early months of 1857 suggested that a major source of *bakufu* opposition to vaccination had been removed.

By this time it was widely recognized that children who had been vaccinated with cowpox vaccine did not get smallpox. As smallpox swept through Japan's northern territories, Muragaki Norimasa, an Ezo official, requested that the *bakufu* send physicians from Edo to vaccinate the people of Ezo against smallpox.[2] In Edo, the Rōjū Abe Masahiro, the *bakufu*'s chief minister, commissioned a medical mission to go to Ezo.[3] This was the *bakufu*'s first official act acknowledging vaccination, but the initiative had come from a local official in Ezo. Unlike the early vaccinations commissioned by Japan's regional lords, the *bakufu*'s directive required little political risk. The officially sanctioned vaccinations in Ezo were directed at the Ainu population living on Japan's northern periphery, a population that was not regarded as Japanese. If vaccination were to cause problems there, the repercussions would take place far from the capital. There were to be no vaccinations, symbolic or otherwise, of Tokugawa offspring or the children of the imperial family.

The Edo *machi bugyō* posted announcements that described the situation in Ezo and asked physicians who were competent to perform vaccination to come forward. In April 1857, the *bakufu* announced that six qualified Edo physicians would be sent to Ezo. Kuwata Ryūsai, Edo's enthusiastic publicist for vaccination, and Fukase Yōshun, an Edo physician originally from Hakodate in Ezo, were chosen to lead the vaccination mission. Like Ryūsai, Fukase Yōshun was an active member of the Edo *ranpō* community. He had previously studied with Itō Genboku, Satō Taizen, and Takenouchi Gendō. The medical mission left Edo with a recently vaccinated child as the initial donor of the cowpox virus. It would recruit other children as donors along the way, in order to keep an effective supply of lymph on hand.

The vaccinators were instructed to include the northernmost islands of Kunashiri, Etorofu, Uruppu, and the southern half of Sakhalin in the territories to be covered, and to vaccinate the Japanese as well as the Ainu inhabitants. Determined to vaccinate as many children as possible, the two doctors divided the Ezo territories between them. Not surprisingly, there was initial resistance and many people fled as the vaccinators approached. Eventually, however, local administrators took control of the operation and required children to report to certain clinics on designated days of the week to be vaccinated. The *bakufu*'s vaccination team spent three months working cooperatively with local Japanese officials and with Ezo's Ainu leaders. When Kuwata Ryūsai and Fukase Yōshun returned to Edo, they claimed to have vaccinated 5,150 children in Ezo and the Tohoku region.[4]

The Tokugawa *bakufu*'s sponsorship of the Ezo expedition suggested that the government's attitude toward vaccination had become more lenient. Edo's *ranpō* physicians decided the time had come to seize the initiative. In July 1857 (Ansei 4.6), a small group of interested physicians gathered at the home of Ōtsuki Shunsai to discuss the preparation of a petition to submit to the Shogun Tokugawa Iesada, asking for permission to open a vaccination clinic in Edo. Although private vaccinations had been performed in doctors' offices and domain *yashiki* for almost a decade, there still was no vaccination clinic in Edo.

In attendance at the June meeting were Itō Genboku, Totsuka Seikai, Takenouchi Gendō, all former students of von Siebold; Hayashi Dōkai, Miyake Gonsai, who were affiliated with Satō Taizen; and four or five other physicians, including Mitsukuri Genpo, the physician employed by the shogun.[5] Ōtsuki Shunsai and Itō Genboku had organized the meeting, but Mitsukuri Genpo was the key person in attendance. All the others were well-established Edo physicians, but their political connections were with various *daimyō* not the Tokugawa government.

Mitsukuri Genpo (1799–1863) was of the same generation as Genboku and Shunsai, a native of Tsuyama domain (Okayama Prefecture). He was the second son of a *kanpō* physician. Genpo had gone to Edo in 1823 to study Western medicine with Udagawa Genshin, also a native of Tsuyama domain. After Genshin's death in 1834, Genpo had opened his own medical practice in Edo, but his health was poor; when a fire destroyed the building where he saw patients, he did not rebuild. Instead, he became a full-time scholar and translator of Dutch books and the editor of *Taisei meii ikō,* Japan's first medical journal mentioned above. Genpo had been an active member of the Shōshikai in the 1830s, and like other members of that group his interests had expanded into fields of inquiry that were not associated with medicine. Like Itō Genboku and Ōtsuki Shunsai, Genpo had escaped the *bakufu*'s purge of 1839, which claimed the lives of other members of the Shōshikai. In fact, it was Mitsukuri Genpo who had replaced Koseki San'ei at the Tenmondai after San'ei's suicide following the 1839 purge.

Mitsukuri Genpo's speciality was the translation of Western books dealing with foreign trade. Despite the fact that he probably knew little, if any, Russian, Genpo was appointed to represent the Edo government as its official interpreter in the trade negotiations with the Russian delegation at Nagasaki in 1853 and Shimoda in 1854. These assignments led to an acquaintance with Kawaji Toshiakira, also a former member of the Shōshikai, who headed the Japanese delegation at these negotiations. During the Russian negotiations, Genpo developed a close relationship with his superior. In 1857, Toshiakira was serving the Tokugawa *bakufu* as Minister of the Treasury (*kanjō bugyō*), one of the three top positions in the Edo government. It was Mitsukuri Genpo's special relationship with Kawaji Toshiakira that made him the key figure at the meeting in Ōtsuki Shunsai's house.[6]

Government ministers had short tenures during this period, and it was essential to move quickly. The physicians met at Ōtsuki Shunsai's house again in the fall to draw up a petition to the Shogun Tokugawa Iesada in the name of Kawaji Toshiakira. The petition requested permission to build a vaccination clinic on a site in Edo's Kanda district, which Toshiakira had offered to donate for this purpose. The petition was granted: it authorized the construction of a vaccination clinic at the Kanda site in front of the Buddhist temple Seigan-ji. The clinic was called the Otamagaike Shutōjo (Otamagaike Vaccination Clinic), and it opened in February 1858.

The *bakufu*'s permission to build this clinic did not extend to financial support for the project. Funds to build and staff the clinic still had to be raised by subscription from private sources, and the organizers already had donors in mind. They quickly produced a list of names of relatives, students, friends, and associates of the organizers. This list, compiled in the hand of Ōtsuki Shunsai, contains the names of eighty-three sponsors of the Otamagaike Shutōjo.

The sponsors of the Otamagaike Vaccination Clinic are regarded as the founding fathers of modern medicine in Japan. By 1858, many of the brightest and most dedicated proponents of vaccination had succumbed to illness or to the repressive policies of the *bakufu*. Those who had survived had been patient: they had learned to focus solely on medicine and to avoid expressing any opinion on political matters. Their long-term strategy—first, to acquire cowpox vaccine and second, to prove the efficacy of vaccination, *before* petitioning the shogun for permission to vaccinate openly in Edo—had paid off. By choosing the successes of vaccination to demonstrate the value of Western medicine, *ranpō* physicians had achieved a strong position from which to influence medical policy at the top levels of government.

The early vaccination promoters, even today, are regarded as benefactors of the Japanese people. Vaccination is viewed as a public benefit, and monuments and institutions honoring Japan's vaccinators can be found in the towns and villages from which they came. Claimed as local as well as national heroes, their homes and schools are preserved as shrines; their writings and effects can be seen in private and public libraries and in museum collections; and the stories of their lives have been reconstructed by scholars and family biographers. The story of Itō Genboku's life, for example, is featured in a comic book that is given to students who attend the local school in Nihiyama.[7]

The importance attached to the early vaccinators in the public mind has meant that Japanese scholars have sought to learn as much as possible about the individuals whose names appear on the Otamagaike sponsorship list. Consequently, a surprising amount of information is known about many of the sponsors. Research on this list has revealed not only the composition of the *ranpō* medical community active in Edo at mid-century; it also reveals the enduring connections between physicians in different parts of Japan and between the different generations within the *ranpō* community.

Table 7.1 lists the names of eighty-three physician sponsors of the Otamagaike Vaccination Clinic as compiled by Ōtsuki Shunsai. The table gives known birth and death years for forty-two of the sponsors. Table 7.1 was compiled with the assistance of Dr. Fukase Yasuaki, a medical historian at Juntendō University, to whom I am indebted for many personal details about the sponsors. Using Japanese names to identify individuals who lived in the nineteenth century is one of the more difficult tasks for historians of Japan. The names on the Otamagaike list are especially difficult because, as we have seen, Japanese physicians changed their names frequently. They changed their surnames when they married or were adopted; they changed their professional names when they found a name they preferred; and, like most Japanese, they were known by different names at different times in their lives. To add yet another difficulty, it was not uncommon for a son to take his father's name as his own when his father retired or died. In such cases, it is essential to know the birth and death years of both the father and the son to establish the identity of either.

Identifying the Otamagaike sponsors confronts all of these challenges. Although the original list was written by Ōtsuki Shunsai, when and how it was compiled are unclear. There is no doubt, however, about the importance of the order in which the names are listed. Age and seniority dictated one's place on the list. Names are not grouped by teacher-student or father-son relationships. With few exceptions, the names of the more senior and more famous *ranpō* physicians are at or near the top of the list, and the names of younger, less-known physicians are toward the end. Mitsukuri Genpo's name is first, followed closely by the names of those who met to formulate the petition to the shogun. Although the transmission of cowpox lymph had required participation on a national scale, the Otamagaike Clinic was an Edo project, and the sponsors were primarily *ranpō* physicians living and working in the city.

The names of four of von Siebold's students—Itō Genboku, Takenouchi Gendō, Totsuka Seikai, and Ishii Sōken—are listed near the top. Considering that more than thirty years had passed since these men had had any contact with their teacher, and that many of von Siebold's students were no longer living, this was remarkably strong representation. Mima Junzō and Minato Chōei, the Edo physicians who had assisted Jan Cock Blomhoff even before von Siebold's arrival in 1823, had died in 1825 and 1838, respectively. Two of von Siebold's most outstanding students, Koseki San'ei and Takano Chōei, had been arrested in the 1839 purge and had taken their own lives in 1839 and 1850, respectively. The botanist Kō Ryōsai had died in Osaka in 1846, Hino Teisai had died in Kyoto in 1850, and Narabayashi Sōken had died in Nagasaki in 1852. The German physician's disciples were dying off quickly, but those who remained were as determined as ever to establish Jennerian vaccination as an accepted medical practice in Japan.

TABLE 7.1

Sponsors of the Otamagaike Clinic, birth and death years, signing order

Mitsukuri Genpo	1799–1863	Katsuragawa Hoshū	1826–1881
Takenouchi Gendō	1795–1870	Kosuge Junsei	
Takasu Shōtei	1814–1902	Ishii Sōken	1796–1861
Nagata Sōken		Iwana Shōzan	
Hayashi Dōkai	1813–1895	Nakamura Seitō	
Ōtsuki Shunsai	1806–1862	Fujii Hōsaku	1815–1864
Miyake Gonsai	1817–1868	Yoshida Shūan	
Tsuboi Shinryō	1823–1904	Shinoda Genjun	
Ota Kensai	1824–1908	Yamada Genrin	
Misawa Ryōeki	1817–1868	Shimamura Teiho	1830–1881
Tsuboi Shindō	1832–1867	Itō Gen'min	
Kawamoto Kōmin	1810–1871	Hotoda Gen'etsu	
Totsuka Seikai	1799–1876	Watanabe Shuntei	
Itō Genboku	1800–1871	Katayama Shūtei	1827–1900
Tezuka Ryōan	?–1877	Minobe Kōan	
Watanabe Eisen		Kure Kōseki	1811–1879
Tezuka Ryōsai	1824–1875	Muraita Genryū	
Totsuka Seiho	1824–1884	Nishikawa Gentai	
Itō Gencho		Kikuchi Kaiju	
Itō Nanyō	1804–1884	Hirano Genkei	
Yamamoto Chōan	1822–1902	Sugano Dōjun	1810–1867
Ōno Shōsai	1819–1888	Makiyama Shūkyō	
Andō Genshō	1817/27–1876	Okuyama Genchū	1810–1905
Masuki Ryōsai		Kawashima Sōtan	
Adachi Baiei		Tamura Taizō	
Kojima Shuntei	1822–1871	Ikeda Tachū	1820–1872
Tsuda Chōshun		Kōsaka Ryōan	
Ishikawa Ōsho	1822–1882	Takahashi Jun'eki	1831–1865
Nonaka Gen'ei		Miura Yūkō	1812–1890
Kuwata Ryūsai	1811–1868	Ōta Tokai	1829–1875
Suzuki Gentai		Mizoguchi Seimin	
Ōta Sessai		Iwai Genkei	
Sugita Gentan	1818–1889	Ayabe Zentatsu	
Akagi Ryōhaku	1797–1884	Masushiro Ryōho	
Matsumoto Ryōho	1806–1877	Ōtsuki Genshun	1841–1908
Sugita Kyōsai		Kawashima Gensei	1827–1873
Soeta Genshun	1800–1860	Ōkuma Ryōtatsu	
Irisawa Teii	1800–1860	Yanagi Kensen	1829–1901
Yoshida Jun'an		Sakakibara Genshin	1844 – ?

Table 7.1 (continued)

Okabe Dōchoku	Ōtaka Genshun
Kobayashi Gendō	Kaida Kōsai
Nogi Bunteki	

SOURCES: *Dankyō shutōjo kifuseimei roku (Record of Official List of Shutōjo Sponsors)*; Itō Sakae, *Itō Genboku den (A Biography of Itō Genboku)* (Tokyo: Genbusha, 1916; reprint, Yashio Shoten, 1978), 94–96; and Fukase Yasuaki. "Otamagaike shutō kaisetsu o megutte" ("A Consideration of the Otamagaike Vaccination Clinic"), Part 2, *Nihon ishigaku zasshi* 26, 4 (1980): 420–421. Supplemented with personal information from Dr. Fukase Yasuaki.

The sponsorship list makes it clear that the physicians who participated in the initial distribution of cowpox vaccine had been able to mobilize younger supporters. Ōtsuki Shunsai's contingent included Tezuka Ryōan and Tezuka Ryōsai, from the family of his teacher and father-in-law, Tezuka Ryōsen. The names of Ōtsuki Shunsai's young son, Ōtsuki Genshun, and Shunsai's student, Ōta Tōkai, by then a relative by marriage, are found near the end of the list. The names of six other individuals known to have been closely associated with Ōtsuki Shunsai are on the sponsorship list as well. Other signers who cannot be identified also may have been associated with him.

At least eight sponsors can be identified as Itō Genboku's students or family members: Ikeda Tachū, Itō Genmin, Kojima Shuntei, Masushiro Ryōho, Nonaka Gen'ei, Kojima Shuntei, Suzuki Gentai, and Yanage Kensen are all are listed in the student register of Shōsendō, Itō Genboku's private academy. Itō Genmin was Genboku's son and Nonaka Gen'ei was an adopted son.[8]

Satō Taizen was no longer practicing medicine in Edo, but he too was well represented by family members and students. The name of Hayashi Dōkai, Taizen's son-in-law and the Director of Wada-juku, is found near the top of the list. Taizen's second son, Matsumoto Ryōjun, and his lifelong friend, Matsumoto Ryōho, who adopted Ryōjun, were both sponsors of the clinic, as was Miyake Gonsai, Taizen's former student and surgical associate at the Juntendō Medical School in Sakura.[9]

Tsuboi Shindō, the teacher who had trained so many *ranpō* physicians at his Edo school, had died in 1848; but his eldest son, Tsuboi Shinyū, his son-in-law, Tsuboi Shinryō, and his former student, Kuwata Ryūsai, are all listed as sponsors. Kuwata Ryūsai must only recently have returned from the intensive vaccination campaign in Ezo when the sponsorship list was being compiled. Tsuboi Shindō's influence was represented also, though indirectly, through his most accomplished student, Ogata Kōan. Kōan was neither an Edo physician nor a sponsor of the Edo clinic, but several of his students' names are on the list of sponsors. Nonaka Gen'ei, Okabe Dōchaku, Tezuka Ryōan, and Tsuboi Shinyū, *ranpō* physicians now living in Edo, were Otamagaike sponsors. One sponsor was the father of Iwana Shōzan, a former student of Ogata Kōan at Tekijuku.[10]

More connections than can be traced today must have existed between the sponsors. This is not surprising. These physicians became sponsors because of their obligations to and associations with one or more of the other signers, as well as because they supported vaccination. But even this small sample emphasizes the extent to which the Edo *ranpō* network incorporated fathers, sons, uncles, nephews, brothers-in-law, sons-in-law, teachers, and students from other parts of Japan. The vaccination network integrated various medical lineages to produce a loosely constructed professional association. The sponsorship list identifies lateral connections which were based on personal and professional loyalties that transcended the political boundaries of domain and office.

Particularly noteworthy is the fact that all the major *ranpō* schools are represented on the list of sponsors. There are no obvious omissions. The Otamagaike Clinic was an inclusive, not an exclusive, venture. Participating physicians recognized the importance of obtaining official recognition for vaccination from the Tokugawa *bakufu*. The sponsors of the clinic whose names appear on Ōtsuki Shunsai's list were all physicians, but Fukase Yasuaki believes that Saitō Genzō, the merchant who dealt in Western medicines, was also a sponsor of the clinic, despite the fact that his name is not on the list. Genzō was present at the first meeting at Ōtsuki Shunsai's house, and he was involved from the outset in the plans for construction of the clinic building. Saitō Genzō was the son of Kanzakiya Genzō, the pharmacist who had come to Edo from Sendai and established the Kanzakiya pharmaceutical firm in the city. The elder Genzō had underwritten the medical educations of Ōtsuki Shunsai and Takano Chōei, and he developed close ties with the Edo *ranpō* community. He died in 1837, but his son, also Saitō Genzō, maintained a close association with the Ōtsuki family, and he continued to support the activities of *ranpō* physicians in Edo. Fukase concludes that Saitō Genzō was a substantial donor to the clinic at Otamagaike.[11]

Tables 7.2 and 7.3 show the composition of the group of sponsors by age and generation, respectively. Calculations of age in Table 7.2 are based on Japanese age (*sai*), because conversions to approximate Western ages would not help clarify the age relationships among the sponsors.

TABLE 7.2

Sponsors of the Otamagaike Clinic by age cohort

Sai (Japanese age)	Number of sponsors	Sai (Japanese age)	Number of sponsors
60 and older	4	30–39	14
50–59	6	20–29	4
40-49	12	Less than 20	2

Sai = the number of Japanese calendar years in which a person has lived. By Western calculation, the individuals could be as much two years younger.

TABLE 7.3

Sponsors of the Otamagaike Clinic by birth decade

Before 1800	1810-1819	1820-1829	1830-1839	1840 and Later
6	12	19	4	2

The age range is 63 to 14 *sai*: Takenouchi Gendō, born in 1795 was the oldest; Sakakibara Genshin and Ōtsuki Shunsai's son, Genshun, both born in 1844, were the youngest. The absence of birth and death year data for half of the sponsors gives an upward bias to the age distribution, because more birth years are known for the older, established physicians whose names are at the top of the list. Birth and death data exist for a much smaller proportion of the presumably younger sponsors whose names are concentrated at the end of the list.

Eleven sponsors would not live to witness the fall of the Tokugawa shogunate and the advent of the Meiji era in 1868, but fifteen would live into the 1880s and seven into the twentieth century. The generational distribution of the sponsors makes it clear that that the senior *ranpō* physicians had prepared the next generation to succeed them. The preponderance of the clinic's sponsors seem to have been below age fifty. These younger physicians would staff not only the Otamagaike Vaccination Clinic but also the soon-to-be-created public health bureaucracy, and some of them would serve on the faculty at the new imperial university in Edo.

Construction of the vaccination clinic at Otamagaike began in early 1858, and the clinic opened in June. Just six months later, it was destroyed in a fire that started at dawn and swept through Kanda.[12] However, the impasse between the vaccinators and the *bakufu* had been broken: The shogun had sanctioned the founding of an Edo vaccination clinic, and permission to rebuild the clinic was not required. Plans to build a new clinic began at once. Within this short period, Tokugawa Iesada had died and Kawaji Toshiakira had fallen from favor. He could not offer assistance a second time, and the physicians who had donated money six months earlier could not do so again. New patrons were forthcoming, however, and this time merchant sponsorship of the new facility is clear: Hamaguchi Goryō, a wealthy Sakura sake merchant, was among those to donate funds to rebuild the clinic. Meanwhile, Ōtsuki Shunsai and Itō Genboku continued to perform vaccinations at their residences, and in September 1859, a new vaccination clinic was opened nearby in Shitaya's Izumibashi-dōri.

The second clinic, like the first, was built with private funds, but not long after it opened the Tokugawa *bakufu* actively began to support vaccination in Edo for the first time. The government gave administrative support to the new clinic and disseminated information and advice about vaccination. On November 26, 1860 (Man'en 1.10.14), the Tokugawa *bakufu* assumed the management of the clinic, reinforced its finances, and appointed Ōtsuki Shunsai to be the clinic's first Director.

Under Ōtsuki's direction, the mission of the clinic expanded and took on the functions of a Western-style medical school. In 1861, the clinic's name was changed to Seiyō Igakusho—Institute of Western Medicine.[13] Physicians who had sponsored the Otamagaike Clinic became the Institute's faculty, and the most senior physicians were given the title of Professor (*kyōjū*). The medical faculty continued to perform vaccinations, but they also taught dissection, autopsy, and other skills considered to be part of a Western medical curriculum. The senior faculty included Itō Genboku, Takenouchi Gendō, and Hayashi Dōkai, none of whom had previously been employees of the *bakufu*. But *bakufu* physicians, such as Matsumoto Ryōho, Katsuragawa Hoshū, and Yoshida Shōan, were also on the faculty. Thus, the Seiyō Igakusho produced a merger of private and public physicians at the very center of Japanese politics. The two groups of *ranpō* physicians had long worked collaboratively, but it was only in the final years of Tokugawa rule that they could do so officially in an explicitly Western-oriented institution under government auspices.

As the elder members of the vaccination network died off, they were replaced by younger members. On May 7, 1862 (Bunkyū 2.4.9), Ōtsuki Shunsai died of stomach cancer, and the *bakufu* summoned Ogata Kōan to Edo to replace him. This summons imposed a great hardship on Kōan who was not well, but he left his family, school, and medical practice in Osaka and came to Edo to take up his new position. He served for little more than a year: Ogata Kōan died of a massive hemorrhage on July 25, 1863 (Bunkyū 3.6.10). Shortly before Kōan's death, on April 2, 1863 (Bunkyū 3.2.5), the *bakufu* changed the name of Seiyō Igakusho to Igakusho—or simply, Medical Institute.[14]

Thus, during a five-year period in which the Tokugawa *bakufu* was besieged with overwhelming internal and external problems, a small group of private physicians was granted permission to found a vaccination clinic on borrowed land in the center of Edo. In short order it had been transformed into a full-fledged Japanese medical school specializing in Western medicine. The private Otamagaike Vaccination Clinic had become a public institution funded by the Tokugawa government. Its new name signified that Western-style medicine no longer needed to be labeled "Western;" it was simply one type of medicine practiced in Japan. Thus, the successes of vaccination had led the way to legitimizing Western-style medicine.

If Japan's *ranpō* physicians had aspired to higher social status, they were well rewarded. Once vaccination advocates established a beachhead in Japan's political center, the Edo government created new official positions that had the responsibility of administering the new institutions. The top positions passed quickly from one member of the vaccination network to another. Senior sponsors of the Otamagaike Clinic held the first administrative and faculty posts at the Seiyō Igakusho, but it was not long before they were replaced by younger members. In 1862, Hayashi Dōkai, age forty-nine, replaced the oldest faculty appointee, Takenouchi Gendō, age sixty-seven. At least thirteen sponsors of the Otamagaike Clinic served in official and faculty positions at the Seiyō Igakusho and its successor institution, the Igakusho. After Ogata Kōan's death, Matsumoto Ryōjun, Satō Taizen's son, became the new Director of the Igakusho.[15]

At the end of the Tokugawa period, *ranpō* physicians held positions of influence at the very apex of the Edo government. In 1861, Itō Genboku had been called to Edo Castle to examine the young Shogun, Tokugawa Iemochi (r. 1858–1866), when the latter suffered an attack of fever.[16] And when two members of the British Legation to Japan were shot and wounded in 1862, Genboku's son, Itō Kansai, was summoned to treat them.[17] Perhaps the most significant sign of Itō Genboku's rise to prominence was his attendance upon the Imperial Princess Kazunomiya when she came from Kyoto to Edo for her marriage to the Shogun Iemochi later that year. During Genboku's medical examination of the princess, Totsuka Seikai, Takenouchi Gendō, Hayashi Dōkai, and Itō Kansai were all in attendance.[18] One can speculate about the role of these witnessing physicians, but, as we have seen, it was not unusual for witnesses to be present when new and unusual medical procedures took place for the first time, as when the English royal children were inoculated in London in the 1700s.

* * *

Even more radical initiatives were developing elsewhere in Japan as the Tokugawa hegemony came to a close. As Edo's *ranpō* physicians were preparing a petition asking the shogun's permission to open a vaccination clinic in the Tokugawa capital, and as the Tokugawa *bakufu* was preparing to send an official mission to vaccinate the children of Ezo, new medical initiatives were already underway in the city of Nagasaki. The *bakufu* had invited Dutch doctors and pharmacists to come to Japan to assist with the opening of a new Western-style medical school; and in November 1857, the Dutch doctor, Johannes Lidius Catharinus Pompe van Meerdervoort, arrived in Nagasaki. Pompe had trained at the Utrecht Medical College in Holland, and he was the first of many foreign medical professionals to participate in building medical institutions during the late Tokugawa and early Meiji periods. The Nagasaki Medical School opened in 1858 with only twelve students, but the number of students at the school grew rapidly as Japan's domain lords, from Kyushu and western Honshu in particular, sent students to study at the new medical school.[19]

At Pompe's request, the *bakufu* authorized the founding of a hospital at Nagasaki, and in September 1861, the Nagasaki Hospital opened as a teaching hospital for the Medical School.[20] These two institutions were models for other Western medical institutions founded later by the Meiji government. The Nagasaki Hospital was a two-story building with 128 beds, built in Western architectural style in the shape of an H.[21] A hospital was an entirely new concept in Japan, and the building itself must have seemed a peculiar intrusion upon the landscape of the city. Traditionally, sick patients had been treated in the homes and clinics of private physicians. The major tasks of this new medical complex were to design a medical program for students studying at the school, and to construct clinical out-patient and in-patient facilities at the hospital to serve both students and the community.

Vaccination services in that area became the responsibility of the Nagasaki medical staff. Pompe wrote that one of his regular tasks at the hospital was vaccinating local children and foreigners coming into the port of Nagasaki on infected ships. Pompe credited his compatriot, Otto Mohnike, with having organized a regular vaccination service in Nagasaki and maintaining a good supply of vaccine, but he claimed that the vaccination program had not been well maintained after Mohnike's departure in 1851. Pompe was hardly in a position to know how well the vaccine was managed elsewhere in Japan, but until the opening of Japan's ports in 1858, importing live vaccine from Batavia remained as difficult as before Mohnike's arrival. Once the ports opened, it was possible to import fresh vaccine from nearby countries in Asia. When a smallpox epidemic broke out in Nagasaki that same year, Pompe could request vaccine from a missionary in China. Apparently vaccine arrived quickly: Pompe claimed to have vaccinated more than 1,300 children in 1858 and 1859.[22]

Shortage of vaccine was not the only problem. One way to assess the effectiveness of vaccination is to consider the consequences of failure to use it. The most striking example is the premature and untimely death of Emperor Kōmei from smallpox in early 1867.[23] Although domain lords began to have their children vaccinated soon after the arrival of vaccine in 1848, the imperial family did not follow suit. The idea of inoculating the Japanese Emperor and other members of the imperial family with a disease of cows was probably beyond consideration. The Emperor's death, so soon after the death in August of the Shogun Tokugawa Iemochi, contributed greatly to the political instability of the period, and it led directly to the early succession of the fifteen-year-old Meiji Emperor.

Meanwhile, developments in Nagasaki opened the way for Japanese physicians to work and study openly with Dutch medical personnel for the first time. Those who went to Nagasaki to study with the foreign doctors during this period would be appointed to the top posts in the Meiji government and form Japan's new medical elite. Descendents of Japan's vaccinators were the first to take advantage of the opportunity to study in Nagasaki. Ogata Kōan's oldest son, Heizō, and Satō Taizen's adopted son and heir, Satō Shōchū, went to Nagasaki to study with Pompe in the late 1850s. And two physicians who had been primed since birth for careers in Western medicine, Matsumoto Ryōjun (Jun), Satō Taizen's second son, and Nagayo Sensai, the grandson of Nagayo Shuntatsu, went to Nagasaki to study with Pompe in 1857 and 1860, respectively.

Matsumoto Jun (1832–1907) was born in Edo shortly before his father, Satō Taizen, went to study in Nagasaki with Hayashi Dōkai. As he would write in his memoirs, he was the first of his siblings to be variolated by his father. Jun seems to have been chosen by his father for special grooming, because in 1849, at age seventeen, he was adopted by Taizen's close friend, the *bakufu* physician, Matsumoto Ryōho. This adoption effectively removed him from the Satō lineage and any claim to succeed to a hereditary position at Juntendō Medical School. Instead, he entered the official Tokugawa system; the same year he passed an entrance examination, which, as Matsumoto Ryōho's son, qualified him to study at the Igakkan.[24] In 1855, at age 23, he became an official Tokugawa doctor,[25] and in 1857 the *bakufu* sent him to Nagasaki to study and work with Pompe.[26]

Matsumoto Jun helped Pompe set up the Nagasaki Medical School and Hospital. He learned dissection from the Dutch physician, and he was still in Nagasaki when Nagayo Sensai arrived in 1860. Jun was called back to Edo after Ogata Kōan's death in 1863 to replace him as Director of the Igakusho, and later he was appointed the first Surgeon General of the Tokugawa army.[27] Matsumoto Jun was well positioned to function within the government as an advocate for medical reform along Western lines, and he seems to have remained a loyal official of the Tokugawa shogunate until the very end. If so, this loyalty did not prevent his becoming a major political and military figure in the Meiji government, which eventually gave him the title of Baron.[28]

Nagayo Sensai (1838–1904), who would become the creator of Japan's public health bureaucracy, had a very different background.[29] He was the grandson of Nagayo Shuntatsu of Ōmura domain, who had read Jenner's treatise in the 1830s and tried to create cowpox virus by inoculating cows with smallpox. When Shuntatsu's experiments proved unsuccessful, he had opened a variolation retreat in the Ōmura mountains, where he inoculated children with the smallpox virus until the cowpox vaccine arrived in 1849.[30]

Shuntatsu had sought a Western-oriented medical education for his grandson, and he sent him to Osaka to study with Ogata Kōan at Tekijuku. Sensai became the top student (*jukutō*) at Tekijuku. Although Sensai planned to go to Edo to study after Osaka, Kōan persuaded him to go to Nagasaki instead, where Kōan's son, Heizō, was already studying with Pompe. In Edo, Kōan said, one could study only Japanized Western medicine; whereas, in Nagasaki, one would have an opportunity to study with the Dutch physicians who were teaching there.[31]

Nagasaki was an excellent place for an ambitious young man to be in the 1860s. The political situation in Edo was unstable as the government struggled with internal factions and external forces. The Tokugawa *bakufu* was going through extremely difficult times: Tokugawa Iesada died in 1858 at age thirty-four, having been shogun for only five years; and his successor, the twenty-year-old Tokugawa Iemochi, a distant cousin, died in 1866.[32] There were no direct descendents in the Tokugawa line, and controversies over a suitable successor from a collateral Tokugawa line caused great dissention. It was advantageous to be somewhere other than Edo during this period.

On December 9, 1867, when the last Tokugawa shogun, Tokugawa Yoshinobu, stepped down, and the young Emperor Meiji moved from Kyoto to Edo, renamed Tokyo at that time, Nagayo Sensai was still in Nagasaki. The Western-oriented Meiji oligarchs who came to power and formed a new national government in Edo appointed Nagayo Sensai the Director of the Nagasaki Medical School and Hospital. Sensai's decision to study and work with the Dutch physicians employed in Nagasaki had paid off.

Nagayo Sensai sought foreign expertise and advice from the very beginning of his career. Pompe was the resident foreign doctor when he arrived in Nagasaki. He taught anatomy by dissection and autopsy, a radical departure from traditional medicine in Japan. Cadavers were not easy to get in Japan, so Pompe ordered a cadaver from Paris so he could personally introduce the techniques of dissection to his students. Antonius Franciscus Bauduin, who came when Pompe left, taught Sensai surgical medicine, and later Cornelius van Mansvelt would advise Sensai on issues related to medical education. It was van Mansvelt who convinced Sensai to begin his medical school reforms by building a premedical program offering students a basic curriculum with courses in mathematics, physics, chemistry, botany, and zoology. The Dutch pharmacist and science teacher Antonie Johannes Cornelis Geertz was put in charge of developing a premedical program at the Nagasaki Medical School.

As Director, Sensai authorized a series of important reforms in the late 1860s, adding anatomy, physiology, and pathology to the Medical School curriculum. He actively engaged the interest and involvement of political figures from western Japan who would become Japan's early Meiji leaders in his educational reforms. For example, he successfully appealed to Inouye Kaoru for funds to buy books and equipment, to hire foreign teachers, and to procure the cadavers of executed criminals needed for dissection.

Nagayo Sensai was called to Tokyo in 1871 to begin the reform of medical education in Japan's new capital city. But as politics were still unsettled there, he decided to apply to the government for permission to go to the United States and Europe as a member of the Iwakura Mission, a fact-finding mission whose members sought useful information about foreign institutions and technology.[33] This was an eye-opening trip for Sensai, and it changed his ideas about what he wanted his life's work to be. While he was in Germany, a nation that like Japan was modernizing and centralizing its government, Sensai became attracted to the sanitary and public health movements developing in Europe at the time:

> I heard the words "sanitary" and "health" everywhere and, in Berlin, "Gesundheitphlege." But I did not really understand these words. Eventually I came to understand that these words meant not only protection of the citizens' health, but referred to an entire administrative system that was being organized to protect the citizens' health—a system that relied not only on medicine but on physics, meteorology, and statistics, a system which operated through state administration to eliminate threats to life and to improve the nation's welfare.[34]

These concepts reached far beyond the concepts of medical practice in Japan, with its focus on individual relationships between doctor and patient. Public health meant draining swamps and providing proper sewage disposal and clean water systems. It meant keeping records to track the incidence of infectious disease; it meant educating the public about proper hygiene. These activities involved not only physicians, but local and central governments. It also meant controlling infectious diseases, which required surveillance, mandatory reporting of disease outbreaks, and the collaboration of departments of police. These activities were well beyond the scope of medical practice. They required a state bureaucracy, which in Japan had yet to be created.

When Nagayo Sensai returned to Japan in 1872, the Meiji government made him Japan's first Director of the new Central Sanitary Bureau (Eisei Kyoku). At about the same time, Matsumoto Jun was made the Head of Military Medicine. From these positions, as heads of the civil and military health bureaucracies, these two men would formulate the aggressive policies that produced a new system of medical education based on Western (primarily German) medicine, and a centralized system of public health controlled by the state.

Matsumoto Jun and Nagayo Sensai were transitional figures who spanned the Tokugawa-Meiji divide. They came of age in an era when medical practice was largely a private affair, when physicians were free to practice as they wished as long as they did not engage in politics critical of the Tokugawa government. With the opening of the country, they and others of their generation moved into the public arena to become bureaucrats of a centralizing Japanese state. Within only a few decades, this state would aggressively be exporting its version of Western-style medicine to its new colonies and to the other countries of East Asia.

*   *   *

What impact did the centralization of government have on smallpox mortality and how did vaccination policies develop within the Meiji government? The successful importation of live cowpox virus and its national dissemination in 1849 was only the first stage in limiting the spread of smallpox and lowering smallpox death rates in Japan. The fact that the first generation of post-Tokugawa political leaders, a large number of whom had been trained as doctors, were strong supporters of Westernization meant that support for vaccination continued and was strengthened.

Nagayo Sensai, whose grandfather had been an early vaccination advocate, was now in charge of setting Japan's vaccination policies. The very earliest activities of the Eisei Kyoku involved collecting smallpox and vaccination data from cities and prefectures, and overseeing the work of local physicians who had been performing vaccinations in Japan for over twenty years.[35] Vaccinations would continue to be performed by local physicians, but vaccine production and distribution, and the responsibility for controlling the spread of smallpox, had passed to the central government. Vaccination, which had been introduced to Japan by personal initiative, had become state policy.

How effective were the government's vaccination policies? One of the first to address this question was A. J. C. Geertz, the Dutch physician who had been hired to teach science at the Nagasaki Medical School. Geertz had received his training in medicine and pharmacology at the Army Medical School in Utrecht, and his work in Nagasaki in the early years of the Meiji government eventually secured him a prominent place in the new national health bureaucracy in Tokyo.[36] In June 1879, Geertz published a letter in *The Japan Weekly Mail* acknowledging the importance of extending central government control over vaccination policy in Japan:

A large number of physicians, both Japanese and foreign have, each in his own immediate neighborhood, contributed their share to the work [of vaccination], but this would never have produced such quick and excellent results, if the system had not been governed and controlled by an able hand. For, although . . . vaccination was in a limited degree practiced in the years before 1874, it was not until that time that there appeared regularity, system, order and control in the matter. To Dr. Nagayo Sensai, the chief of the Central Sanitary Office, under the Naimusho [Home Ministry], by far the largest share of praise is incontestably due.[37]

Vaccination policy was the cornerstone of public health policy from the outset. One of Nagayo Sensai's first acts as Director of the Central Sanitary Bureau was to issue a Vaccination Proclamation requiring all children to be vaccinated between 75 and 100 days after birth. All vaccinating physicians had to be certified by the government, and vaccinations were free of charge. Vaccination lesions were to be inspected and certified with a red stamp on an official document. Unsuccessful vaccinees had to be revaccinated and even successful vaccinees had to be revaccinated seven years later. Physicians were required to keep records of the sex and age of vaccinees and to report these statistics to the government every six months. National vaccination statistics were published annually in the *Eisei kyoku nenpō* (*Annual Report of the Central Sanitary Bureau*).[38]

One of the first steps in bringing "regularity, system, order and control" to the matter was extending the surveillance of the central government over Japan's many political jurisdictions. In 1875, the Central Sanitary Bureau published the first vaccination statistics from ten cities; total vaccinations were classified as successful vaccinations, unsuccessful vaccinations, and revaccinations. A decade later, the Meiji government's vaccination policies would extend directly into each Japanese household. The new health regulations of 1885 required all citizens to register vaccination results in the *koseki*, the official household registers of the Meiji state. Physicians were required to issue a vaccination certificate to each person vaccinated, and to report to the government the names and addresses of those who had been vaccinated each month. The police were authorized to check on the birth and vaccination certificates of all individuals living in their jurisdictions. New smallpox cases prompted a visit from a local police officer who would determine whether there were unvaccinated children in the family or neighborhood.[39]

Can one assess whether these draconian regulations of the Meiji government had an impact on smallpox morbidity and mortality rates? They were far more extensive and intrusive than vaccination regulations in most other countries at the time. Regional data from mountain villages in central Japan indicate a sharp and permanent decline in child mortality in the age cohort at greatest risk (birth to ten years) after 1885. And the spiking mortality pattern typical of smallpox flattened out as vaccination procedures were enforced and standardized around the country.[40]

National smallpox and vaccination data also show a gradual decline in the number of cases and deaths from smallpox over the next quarter-century. Smallpox deaths were reported to the government every six months from every prefecture after 1885. Serious epidemic years were 1886 with 73,337 cases, 18,676 deaths (case fatality rate, 25 percent); 1893 with 41,898 cases, 11,852 deaths (case fatality rate, 28 percent; 1897 with 41,946 cases, 12,276 deaths (case fatality rate, 29 percent), and 1905 with 10,704 cases, 3,245 deaths (30 percent).[41] It should be noted that the case fatality rate did not fall but rose slightly. The case fatality rate remained within the normal range of 25–30 percent that had been attributed to smallpox for centuries. Smallpox could not be cured; it had to be prevented.

In the early years of Meiji administration, efforts to contain smallpox became part of a much more extensive agenda to control the spread of other serious infectious diseases. The opening of Japan's ports in 1858 effectively ended Japan's *cordon sanitaire* as Japan immediately was exposed to what are called the *bakumatsu* (end of the *bakufu*) epidemics. A surge of new and old diseases launched a quarter-century of high incidence and heightened mortality caused by infectious disease. New diseases like bubonic plague, epidemic typhus, and cholera raged in the late 1850s and 1860s. And a devastating epidemic of measles, which previously had come only sporadically to Japan, struck Japan with devastating consequences in 1862. The most recent epidemic of measles had been thirty years earlier; everyone under the age of 30 was susceptible to measles, and mortality was exceptionally high.[42] Building Japan's herd immunity to new and old diseases, which were establishing new patterns, would take several decades. In the meantime, descendents of the *ranpō* physicians who had staunchly promoted vaccination were creating a public health regime that would eventually rank second to none in its ability to control the spread of disease and lower mortality rates in Japan.

A movement that had begun in severely limited circumstances on Japan's far periphery had moved to center stage. It had, in fact, moved beyond center stage. Japan's public health initiatives quickly moved into the world beyond Japan. In addition to building a strong public health regime at home, Japan joined the international health initiatives that were developing at the time.

The Meiji government sent official representatives to the International Sanitary Conferences, which, beginning in the 1850s, became an important international forum for limiting the spread of disease across national borders. And Japanese physicians were sent to Europe to learn about Western medicine directly. The timing of Japan's entry onto the world stage was fortuitous: Japanese researchers were soon contributing to the bacteriological revolution—based on the discovery of the germ theory of disease—that was just around the corner.

Conclusion

What does this lengthy narrative tell us about the impact of medical knowledge on the opening of Japan? Focusing on the activities of a generation of physicians who took up the practice of Western medicine and mobilized support for Jennerian vaccination, this book claims that the process of importing this new technology, exceedingly slow and fraught with difficulties, created a new social and intellectual elite during the first half of the nineteenth century. This new elite comprised groups that operated first at the far periphery of Tokugawa society—*rangaku* scholars, *ranpō* physicians, and Dutch interpreters. It survived the fall of the Tokugawa house to take a central role in creating the political, social, and intellectual infrastructure of the modern Japanese state.

The half-century delay in bringing cowpox vaccine to Japan demonstrates the extreme isolation of the Tokugawa government from the concerns of Japanese society, as well as from important knowledge in the world beyond Japan at the beginning of the nineteenth century. Internal structural barriers prevented useful information from reaching an informed authority that was competent and willing to act upon it. It is in this sense that Japan was a "closed" country. It is in this sense that the physicians featured in this book played a significant role in "opening" the country. *The Vaccinators* views Japan's *ranpō* physicians as important agents of change. What were these changes for Japan, and what were the consequences for those who inadvertently set them in motion?

The *ranpō* physicians whose lives are closely examined here were neither dissidents nor social reformers. There is no evidence that they advocated the fall of the Tokugawa house or that they opposed the rule of the feudal lords whom they served. Rather, they relied on traditional social strategies— education, adoption, and marriage—to build a web of connections that would advance their own social and economic status in Tokugawa society. However, the kinds of connections sought by Japan's *ranpō* physicians transcended the vertical structures of lineage and domain which were fundamental to the Tokugawa system of governance. The study of foreign languages and foreign texts, necessary to the practice of Western-style medicine, took them beyond the frames of reference that were common to Tokugawa society. This special expertise granted *rangaku* scholars and *ranpō* physicians unique standing within the larger society. They had to depend upon one another to solve problems of common interest, and the social and quasi-professional networks they formed were fundamentally horizontal in nature.

Real and fictive lineage ties connected the members of this network across time and space. Focusing on the construction of Japan's vaccination network makes it possible to see how a small group of medical scholars, dedicated to preventing smallpox deaths, expanded over three generations to become an influential national network. Creating this network incurred high social costs. The *ranpō* physicians whose lives are discussed here lived a full life span, but the lives of many of their colleagues were cut short in the purges of the Edo government. The talents of *ranpō* physicians who failed to stay out of trouble politically were lost to society. Moreover, Japan's failure to reap the considerable benefits of vaccination many decades earlier resulted in the needless loss of life to smallpox—20 percent of all children born over a half-century.

Foreign medical texts were the major source of knowledge coming from the West until the 1860s, when the opening of Japan's ports brought many foreigners to Japan for the first time. One could not expect foreign news that arrived informally or by word of mouth to be well received, so it is not surprising that news of vaccination, brought by an anonymous messenger in

1803, attracted no attention. What is surprising is that the significance of vaccination was noted, remembered, and later acted upon by a young Nagasaki interpreter.

The time-honored way for foreign information to reach Japan was through texts, not oral communication. Chinese medical texts had been a major source of medical knowledge for centuries, and after 1800 the Japanese had access to a wide range of imported European medical and scientific texts as well. Dutch books were the most important source of education for Japan's *rangaku* scholars and *ranpō* physicians, and the titles of many of these books can be seen in the bills of lading from the Dutch ships that regularly came to Japan. However, not all books that reached Japan are found on those lists. Neither Jenner's *Inquiry* nor Goldschmidt's book, which discussed Jenner's thesis, is found on extant bills of lading; yet Nagayo Shuntatsu had read the former by 1830, and Mima Junzō and Minato Chōan had already read the latter when they assisted Jan Cock Blomhoff with his vaccination trials in 1823.

The dynamics of the Dutch book trade are not well known, but it is clear that a system of exchange had been worked out between certain Nagasaki interpreters and Dutch merchants. This book trade was the key to maintaining a flow of foreign information to Japan, and an understanding of the mechanics of this quasi-clandestine system might reveal a great deal about other private networks that were responding to foreign stimuli in Japan during the early nineteenth century.

The Vaccinators establishes the translation of Dutch medical books as a major carrier of Western knowledge to Japan. The serious training of Nagasaki interpreters as translators of Dutch medical books began in the eighteenth century, and this skill was passed on to physicians and other scholars interested in the West. The publication of *Kaitai shinsho* (1774), and the *Haruma wage* (1796) by *rangaku* scholars in Edo, fostered greater interest in Western medicine among Japanese physicians elsewhere, and encouraged wider study of the Dutch language for the express purpose of translating Western medical books. During the 1820s, Dutch interpreters and physicians in and around Nagasaki were teaching private students from as far away as Sendai, and private academies in Japan's major cities were enrolling students whose studies emphasized Western learning and the translation of Dutch writings.

Translating Dutch medical books became a cottage industry, and it was an important social as well as intellectual activity. Lineage structures that were the bedrock of Japanese society encouraged collaboration between scholars and produced long-term, cumulative research projects. It was not uncommon for physicians to translate different parts of the same book, to borrow books from one another, to write prefaces for one another, or to seek opinions from other scholars about their translations. Translation projects produced social networks: they created the kinds of connections that led to broad participation in the diffusion of cowpox vaccine in 1849, and eventually to position and prestige in the late Tokugawa and early Meiji bureaucracies.

There can be no question about the importance of the Dutch presence in Japan as a bridge to foreign knowledge. The Dutch court journey from Nagasaki and Edo established a regular conduit through which information could flow between these two cities and to other regions of Japan. By authorizing the presence of a community of Dutch merchants at Nagasaki in the early seventeenth century, the Tokugawa *bakufu* intended to gain access to important foreign information. By isolating the Dutch merchants on the tiny island of Dejima and limiting access to them to its own employees, the *bakufu* intended to establish a monopoly over this foreign information. Knowledge was tribute to be paid by the Dutch to the Tokugawa shogun in exchange for trade.

These policies failed because the Edo government lost touch with which kinds of foreign information might be important; while the Nagasaki interpreters and local officials, who interacted with the Dutch Factory employees on a regular basis, became the exclusive repository of foreign knowledge. The value of the Dutch presence accrued to those who established connections with this repository. While it is difficult to calculate the influence of personal meetings between the Dutch and the *rangaku* scholars at the Edo Nagasakiya, there can be little doubt that these visits made a strong impression on the Japanese. This was especially true after Japanese scholars developed proficiency in the Dutch language. The long tenures of Hendrik Doeff and Jan Cock Blomhoff, and the activism of Philipp Franz von Siebold, were clearly important as well. All three men engaged in collaborative projects with the Japanese, and these projects had long-term consequences. Von Siebold's teachings at Narutaki were a catalyst for Western medical studies in Japan, making it possible for his dedicated students to procure the most useful and up-to-date European medical texts.

Western historians have been far less willing than the Japanese to acknowledge the significant contributions of the Dutch and of Japan's *rangaku* scholars to Japan's rapid modern transformation. Grant Kohn Goodman has argued that Japan's *rangaku* scholars had little impact on Japan's subsequent development. These men, he claims, took little notice of the fact that many of the books they translated had been written much earlier; moreover, they had little interest in the history of Western scientific ideas or scientific experimentation. Goodman concludes that these men contributed little to Japan's understanding of Western science.[1]

This argument holds weight if one focuses on the first generation of Dutch physician-translators, who had few ways to learn about the contexts of the texts that came into their possession; but this was no longer true after 1820. *Ranpō* physicians were requesting recently published European books written by prominent clinical practitioners and translating them in the special schools they established throughout Japan. Japanese physicians were also showing considerable interest in medical experimentation. More than one physician tried to produce cowpox vaccine by inoculating cows with smallpox matter; others experimented with different methods of variolation to determine how best to modify and attenuate the smallpox virus. It was Japanese physicians whose experiments compared Chinese-style and Western-style variolation, and led them to the discovery that cowpox crusts remained viable longer than cowpox lymph. This observation led, in turn, to the innovative idea of importing cowpox crusts instead of lymph from Batavia, and to the breakthrough that brought Jenner's cowpox vaccine to Japan after thirty years of failure. This was not received knowledge but deduction based on experimentation, not unlike Jenner's observations and experiments with the cowpox virus a half-century earlier. Knowledge of the history of Western science would have been of no help whatsoever with this practical task.

The fact that the Tokugawa *bakufu*'s attempt to maintain a monopoly over foreign knowledge had backfired did not go unrecognized by the Edo government. The establishment of the Bureau for the Translation of Barbarian Books in Edo in 1811, in the aftermath of the Russian attacks on Ezo and the Kurile Islands, was an attempt to reassert government control over Western knowledge by bringing Japan's *rangaku* scholars to Edo, and into the Tenmondai, an established government institution.

But it was too late. By 1811, the scholars summoned to Edo to work on translations of Dutch books for the government held an unassailable position. They might be purged for their thoughts and their actions, but they constituted a powerful scholarly community because of their exclusive access to medical and scientific knowledge. They were the only ones who knew enough to determine which books the Bureau for the Translation of Barbarian Books should acquire and translate. The Tenmondai assumed an important transitional role as a quasi-official research institution in the late Tokugawa period, and its personnel, projects, and influence deserve more scholarly attention than they have received thus far.

At mid-century, a new institution would also play an important transitional role by bringing privately held medical knowledge to the government and to the public. The founding of the Otamagaike Vaccination Clinic by private physicians in 1857 was the initial step in the creation of Japan's modern university system. Websites of today's University of Tokyo trace its origins to two Tokugawa institutions—the Tenmondai and the Otamagaike Clinic.[2] They show the Tokyo Imperial University Medical School as a direct descendent of the Vaccination Clinic, and they cite the names of the *ranpō* physicians discussed above as its founders. In similar fashion, the Osaka University Medical School traces its lineage back to the Osaka Jotōkan, the Osaka Vaccination Clinic opened at Tekijuku by Ogata Kōan in 1849. Whether these modern institutions are the true descendents or whether they were adopted at some point along the way, it is clear that Japan's top academic institutions regard Japan's vaccinators as worthy ancestors.

The Vaccinators has presented Jennerian vaccination as a transformative technology with the power to attract followers, forge networks, and create new institutions on its behalf. The high demand for a technology that could prevent a devastating and universal disease, and the short supply of the only agent capable of meeting this demand, combined to give vaccination its power. In Japan, the power of vaccination to attract followers, forge networks, and create new institutions was reinforced by the degree of difficulty involved in acquiring the essential agent, *V. vaccinae*, the cowpox virus for Jenner's vaccine. It was *knowledge* of the benefits of vaccination, not the technology itself, which created a committed following that grew to become national in scope.

The *cordon sanitaire,* which had protected Japan from foreign diseases and limited its access to foreign knowledge for centuries, was breached with the opening of Japan's ports in 1858, but Japan's vaccinators had left a legacy that would help Japan control a major influx of acute infectious diseases. They had shown that sharing knowledge, resources, and personnel was beneficial; that evidence of successes and failures must be collected, stored, and open to scrutiny; and that the public's health was an important element of national power. Western medicine and public health would indeed become an element of national power in Japan in the decades to come. As the germ theory of disease gained acceptance throughout the world in the late nineteenth and early twentieth century, Japan would become an exporter of medical knowledge to the other countries of East Asia.

Japanese Names Mentioned in the Text, with Birth and Death Years

Abe Masahiro	阿部正弘	1819–1857
Adachi Chōshun	足立長儁	1775–1837
Adachi San'ai	足立左内	1778–1845
Baba Sajūrō (Sadayoshi)	馬場佐十郎	1787–1822
Baba Tamehachirō (Sadatsune)	馬場為八郎	1769–1838
Fukase Yōshun	深瀬洋春	?
Hayashi Dōkai	林洞海	1813–1895
Hino Teisai	日野鼎哉	1797–1850
Hotta Masayoshi	堀田正睦	1810–1864
Ishii Sōken	石井宗謙	1796–1861
Itō Genboku	伊東玄朴	1800–1871
Itō Keisuke	伊藤圭介	1803–1901
Kasahara Hakuō (Ryūsaku)	笠原白翁	1809–1880
Katsuragawa Hoken	桂川甫賢	1797–1845
Katsuragawa Hoshū {1}	桂川甫周	1754–1809

Katsuragawa Hoshū [2]	桂川甫周	1826–1881
Kawaji Toshiakira	川路聖謨	1801–1868
Kō Ryōsai	高良齋	1799–1846
Koseki San'ei	小関三栄	1787–1839
Kuwata Ryūsai	桑田立斉	1811–1868
Matsudaira Yoshinaga (Keiei)	松平慶永	1828–1890
Matsumoto Ryōho	松本良甫	1806–1877
Matsumoto Ryōjun	松本良順	1832–1907
Mima Junzō	美馬順三	1795–1825
Minato Chōan	湊長安	1786–1838
Mitsukuri Genpo	箕作阮甫	1799–1863
Miyake Gonsai	三宅艮斎	1817–1868
Narabayashi Eiken	楢林栄建	1801–1875
Narabayashi Sōken	楢林宗建	1803–1852
Nabeshima Naomasa	鍋島直正	1814–1871
Nagayo Sensai	長與専斎	1838–1902
Nagayo Shuntatsu	長與俊達	1791–1855
Naka Ten'yū	中天遊	1783–1835
Nakagawa Jun'an	中川淳安	1739–1786
Ogata Kōan	緒方洪庵	1810–1863
Ogata Shunsaku	緒方春朔	1748–1810
Ōtsuki Gentaku	大槻玄澤	1757–1827
Ōtsuki Shunsai	大槻俊斎	1804–1862
Saitō Genzō (father and son)	斎藤源蔵	?
Satō Taizen	佐藤泰然	1804–1872
Satō Tōsuke	佐藤藤佐	1775–1846
Shizuki Tadao	志筑忠雄	1760–1806
Sugita Genpaku	杉田玄白	1733–1817
Takahashi Kageyasu (Sakuzaemon)	高橋景保	1785–1829
Takano Chōei	高野長英	1804–1850
Tezuka Ryōsen	手塚良仙	? –1877
Takenouchi Gendō	竹内玄同	1805–1880
Taki Motokata	多紀元堅	1795–1857
Tokugawa Iemochi	徳川家茂	1846–1866
Tokugawa Ienari	徳川家斉	1773–1841
Tokugawa Yoshimune	徳川吉宗	1684–1751

Tokugawa Yoshinobu (Keiki)	徳川慶喜	1837–1913
Totsuka Seikai	戸塚静海	1799–1876
Tsuboi Shindō	坪井信道	1795–1848
Udagawa Genshin	宇田川玄真	1769–1835
Udagawa Genzui	宇田川玄随	1755–1797
Udagawa Yōan	宇田川榕庵	1798–1846
Yoshio Chūjirō	吉雄忠次郎	1788–1833
Yoshio Gonnosuke	吉雄権之助	1785–1831
Yoshio Kōgyū (Kōzaemon)	吉雄耕牛	1724–1800

SOURCES: *Asahi Nihon rekishi jinbutsu jiten.* Tokyo:Asahi shinbun sha, 1994; *Yōgaku shi jiten*; Numata, 182-189.

Philipp Franz Von Siebold's Students at Narutaki

Physicians		Sai*	Physicians		Sai*
Aoki Kenzō	青木研蔵	11	Kodama Junzō	児玉順蔵	18
Aoki Shūsuke	青木周	26	Koseki San'ei	小関三英	37
Harada Tanehiko	原田種彦	40	Kurokawa Ryōan	黒川良安	?
Hatazaki Tei	幡崎鼎	17	Kudō Kendō	工藤謙同	23
Hidaka Ryōdai	日高涼台	27	Mima Junzō	美馬順三	30
Hino Teisai	日野鼎哉	27	Minato Chōan	湊長安	30
Honma Genchō	本間玄調	20	Mizuno Genhō	水野玄鳳	26
Hyakutake Banri	百武萬里	30	Morita Sen'an	森田千庵	23
Ishii Sōken	石井宗謙	28	Narabayashi Eiken	楢林栄建	23
Ishizaka Sōki	石坂桑亀	36	Narabayashi Sōken	楢林宗建	22
Itō Genboku	伊東玄朴	24	Narabayashi Sōken	楢林宗建	22
Itō Keisuke	伊藤圭介	21	Ninomiya Keisaku	二宮敬作	20
Itō Shōchū	伊東昇廸	20	Nishi Dōboku	西道朴	64
Kaku Saichirō	賀来佐一郎	23	Oka Kenkai	岡研介	25
Kashiwabara Kenkō	柏原謙好	16	Oka Taian	岡泰安	29
Kō Ryōsai	高良齋	25	Ōtsuka Dōan	大塚同庵	29

Physicians		Sai*	Interpreters		Sai*
Shibata Hōan	柴田方庵	24	Araki Bunkichi	荒木豊吉	?
Suzuki Shūichi	鈴木周一	?	Inabe Ichigorō	稲部市五郎	38
Takano Chōei	高野長英	20	Nakayama Sakusaburō	中山作三郎	39
Takenouchi Gendō	竹内玄同	29	Nishi Keitarō	西慶太郎	?
Taketani Genryū	武谷元立	39	Shige Dennoshin	茂傳之進	?
Totsuka Seikai	戸塚静海	25	Shige Tokijirō	茂土岐次郎	?
Watanabe Kōzō	渡辺幸造	?	Todoroki Takeshichirō	轟武七郎	?
Artist		Sai*	Yoshio Chūjirō	吉雄忠次郎	36
Kawahara Keiga	川原慶賀	38	Yoshio Gonnosuke	吉雄権之助	39
			Yoshio Kōsai	吉雄幸載	36

*Japanese age in 1823.
SOURCES: Kure Shūzō, *Shiiboruto sensei: sono shōgai oyobi kōgyō*. Tokyo, Meicho Kankōkai, 1979, 35-37.

Alphabetized List of Otamagaike Sponsors

Position on
List in
Table 7.1

25	Adachi Baiei	足立梅栄	50	Itō Gen'min	伊東玄民
34	Akagi Ryōhaku	赤城良伯	20	Itō Nanyō	伊東南洋
23	Andō Genshō	安藤玄昌	71	Iwai Genkei	岩井元敬
72	Ayabe Zentatsu	綾部善達	43	Iwana Shōzan	岩名昌山
45	Fujii Hōsaku	藤井方策	83	Kaida Kōsai	甲斐田考斉
5	Hayashi Dōkai	林洞海	53	Katayama Shūtei	片山秀亭
59	Hirano Genkei	平野元敬	40	Katsuragawa Hoshū (2)	桂川甫周
51	Hotoda Gen'etsu	程田玄悦	12	Kawamoto Kōmin	河本幸民
65	Ikeda Tachū	池田多仲	75	Kawashima Gensei	河島元成
38	Irisawa Teii	入沢貞意	63	Kawashima Sōtan	河島宗端
42	Ishii Sōken	石井宗謙	58	Kikuchi Kaijun	菊池海準
28	Ishikawa Ōsho	石川桜所	80	Kobayashi Gendō	小林玄同
14	Itō Genboku	伊東玄朴	26	Kojima Shuntei	小島俊貞
19	Itō Genchō	伊東玄晁	66	Kōsaka Ryōan	上坂良庵

Position on
List in
Table 7.1

41	Kosuge Junsei	小菅純盛
55	Kure Kōseki	呉黄石
30	Kuwata Ryūsai	桑田立斉
73	Masushiro Ryōho	益城良甫
61	Makiyama Shūkyō	牧山修卿
24	Masuki Ryōsai	益木良斉
35	Matsumoto Ryōho	松本良甫
54	Minobe Kōan	美濃部浩庵
10	Misawa Ryōeki	三沢良益
1	Mitsukuri Genpo	箕作元甫
68	Miura Yūkō	三浦有恒
6	Miyake Gonsai	三宅艮斉
70	Mizoguchi Seimin	溝口聖民
56	Muraita Genryū	村板玄竜
4	Nagata Sōken	永田宗見
44	Nakamura Seitō	中村静濤
57	Nishikawa Gentai	西川玄泰
81	Nogi Bunteki	乃木文迪
29	Nonaka Gen'ei	野中玄英
79	Okabe Dōchoku	岡部同直
62	Okuyama Genchū	奥山玄仲
76	Ōkuma Ryōtatsu	大熊良達
22	Ōno Shōsai	大野松斉
32	Ōta Sessai	太田拙斉
69	Ōta Tokai	太田東海
82	Ōtaka Genshun	大高元俊
74	Ōtsuki Genshun	大槻玄俊
6	Ōtsuki Shunsai	大槻俊斉

9	Ota Kensai	織田研斉
78	Sakakibara Genshin	榊原玄辰
49	Shimamura Teiho	島村鼎甫
47	Shinoda Genjun	篠田元順
37	Soeta Genshun	添田玄春
60	Sugano Dōjun	菅野道順
33	Sugita Gentan	杉田玄端
36	Sugita Kyōsai	杉田杏斉
31	Suzuki Gentai	鈴木玄岱
67	Takahashi Jun'eki	高橋順益
3	Takasu Shōtei	高須松亭
2	Takenouchi Gendō	竹内玄同
64	Tamura Taizō	田村泰造
15	Tezuka Ryōan	手塚良庵
17	Tezuka Ryōsai	手塚良斉
18	Totsuka Seiho	戸塚静甫
13	Totsuka Seikai	戸塚静海
8	Tsuboi Shinryō	坪井信良
11	Tsuboi Shindō	坪井信道
27	Tsuda Chōshun	津田良春
16	Watanabe Eisen	渡辺栄仙
52	Watanabe Shuntei	渡辺春汀
48	Yamada Genrin	山田元琳
21	Yamamoto Chōan	山本長安
77	Yanagi Kensen	柳見仙
39	Yoshida Jun'an	吉田淳庵
46	Yoshida Shūan	吉田収庵

Glossary

bakufu	A tent or military government; the Tokugawa government in Edo.
bakumatsu	The end of the *bakufu;* refers to the final decade of the Tokugawa period.
Bansho wage goyō	蛮書和解御用 Bureau for the Translation of Barbarian Books; located in Edo in the Tenmondai.
Batavia	The colonial capital and port city in the Dutch East Indies' island of Java.
bugyō	Tokugawa official, commissioner.
byō	Seed, infective agent; Japanese term used for the smallpox or cowpox virus or lymph.
Chelius	セリウス (Seriusu), *katakana* spelling of M. J. Chelius's surname.
Dejima	A small artificial island in Nagasaki Bay, constructed to serve as a Dutch trading post and residence for Dutch Factory merchants; also pronounced Deshima.
daimyō	Regional overlords of fiefs granted by the shogun; approximately 250 territorial lords held fiefs during the Tokugawa period.

domain	Land held in fief by regional *daimyō* under the Tokugawa shoguns.
Doeff haruma	ツーフハルマ辞書 The Dutch-Japanese dictionary compiled by Hendrik Doeff and selected Dutch interpreters at Dejima in Nagasaki; also called *Dōyaku haruma* 道訳ハルマ, and *Nagasaki haruma* 長崎ハルマ. It was modeled on the Dutch-French dictionary by François Halma.
Dutch Factory	The Dutch trading post on the island of Dejima, 1641–1846.
Edo	The largest castle town in Tokugawa Japan; the site of the military government under the Tokugawa shoguns.
Eisei Kyoku	衛生局 The Central Sanitary Bureau established by the Meiji government in 1873.
Ezo	Northern Japanese island, today's Hokkaidō.
Gyūtō hatsumō	牛痘発蒙 (*Overcoming Ignorance About Smallpox*), by Kuwata Ryūsai, 1849.
"Gyūtō mondō"	牛痘問答 A manuscript on vaccination by Kasahara Hakuō, 1850.
Gyūtō shinsho	牛痘新書 (A new book about cowpox), translation of H. J. Goldschmidt's *Algemeene beschouwing van de geschiedenis der koepokken* . . . Amsterdam, 1802, by Arima Setsuzō, published posthumously in 1850.
Gyūtō shokō	牛痘小考 (About Cowpox), by Narabayashi Sōken, published in Nagasaki, in 1849.
Gyūtō shutō	牛痘種痘 Inoculation with cowpox virus; vaccination.
Haruma wage	波留麻和解 (Japanese translation of François Halma's *Neder-duits woordenboek*, Amsterdam, 1729), Edo, 1796. Also called *Edo haruma*.
Hatamoto	A direct vassal of the Tokugawa shogun.
Hufeland	フヘランド (Huherando), *katakana* spelling of C. W. Hufeland's surname.
Igakkan	医学監 The Tokugawa Medical College in Edo.
inenting	Inoculation, variolation, vaccination (Dutch).
Intō shinpō zensho	印痘新法全書 (*A Complete Book on the New Method of Inoculation*), a Japanese book based on the Chinese text *Yin dou lue*, edited by Koyama Shisei, 2 vols., 1843.
Intō yō ryakkai	印痘要略解 (*A Short Commentary on Vaccination*), by Kuwata Ryūsai, 1849.
Isō kinkan	医宗金鑑 Japanese reading of Chinese title *Yi zong jin jian*.
jintō sesshu	Implanting human pox; variolation.

jintō shutō	人痘種痘 Inoculation with smallpox virus; variolation.
juku	A private academy.
jukutō	The top student in a private academy.
Juntendō	順天堂 Western medical school, founded by Satō Taizen at the invitation of Hotta Masayoshi, *daimyō* of Sakura domain. Today Juntendō Medical School is in Ochanomizu, Tokyo.
kaikoku	Open country; the opening of Japan to the world.
Kaitai shinsho	解体新書 (*New book on anatomy*), a published translation (1774) by Maeno Ryōtaku and Sugita Genpaku of Johann Adam Kulmus's *Anatomischen Tabellen* (1722).
Kangxi	Manchu Emperor of China (r. 1662–1722).
kanbun	Japanese-style Chinese script used for Japanese official documents, medical treatises, many classical texts, and other important writings.
kanjō bugyō	An Edo high government offiicial.
kanpō	漢方 Chinese medical practices.
katakana	A Japanese script used to write foreign words.
kinderpokjes	Smallpox (Dutch).
ko-tsūji	A junior Nagasaki interpreter.
machi bugyō	Tokugawa-appointed city administrators for Edo, Osaka, Kyoto, and Nagasaki.
Matsumae	An Ezo domain held in fief from the Tokugawa shogun by the Matsumae clan.
Miako	The Dutch spelling of Japanese *miyako*; refers to Japan's capital city, Kyoto, where the Japanese Emperors lived until 1868.
Most	モスト (Mosuto), *katakana* spelling of G. F. Chelius's surname.
moxibustion	An ancient form of heat therapy used in East Asia.
Nagasakiya	長崎屋 The official residence where Dutch Factory employees were housed during their stay in Edo.
Narutaki	鳴滝 The Western medical school founded by Philipp Franz von Siebold near Nagasaki, 1823.
Nihongi	日本紀 *Chronicles of Japan: From Earliest Times to 697*. A compilation of Japan's early history, first published in 712.
ō-tsūji	A senior Nagasaki interpreter.
Oppermeester	A physician at Dutch Factory.
Opperhoofd	Director of the Dutch Factory at Dejima.
Pakhuismeester	The warehouse Supervisor at the Dutch Factory.
rangaku	Dutch (Western) learning; refers to Japanese scholarship on Western books.

Rango kanriji kō	蘭語冠履辞考 (*About Dutch Articles*), Baba Sajūrō, 1808.
Rango shubi sesshi kō	蘭語首尾接詞考 (*About Dutch Prefixes and Suffixes*), Baba Sajūrō.
ranpō	蘭方 Literally, Dutch method; Western medical practices.
Rekishō shinsho	暦所新書 (*New Book on Astronomy*), Shizuki Tadao, 1802.
Rōjū	A member of the shogun's Council of Elders.
Roshia gyūtō zensho	露西亜牛痘全書 (*A Russian Book About Smallpox*), Toshimitsu Sen'an's edited edition of Baba Sajūrō's "Tonka hiketsu,"1850.
ryū	流 Literally, current or stream; a school of thought or practices that follow the teachings of a master.
sai	歳 Age, based on number of Japanese calendar years.
Scriba	The Secretary at the Dutch Factory.
Seimi kaisō	舎密開宗 (*Foundations of Chemistry*), by Udagawa Yōan, 1837.
Seisetsu naika senyō	西説内科撰要 (*Selections from Western Medicine*). Udagawa Genzui, 1793.
Senkyō roku	戦競録 Diary of Kasahara Hakuō, October 1849 to 1853; gives an account of the transmission of cowpox vaccine from Kyoto to Fukui.
Shintei gyūtō kihō	新訂牛痘奇法 (*A Newly Revised Edition of the Cowpox Method*), by Hirose Genkyō, 1850.
shogun	The title held by military rulers of Japan after 1185.
shogunate	Japanese military government.
Shōsendō	象先堂 The private academy founded by Itō Genboku in Edo in 1833.
Shōshikai	尚歯会 The research association formed in the 1830s by scholars, physicians, and officials interested in Dutch studies. Prominent members were arrested in the *bakufu* purge of 1839.
Shunzhi	Manchu Emperor of China (r. 1644–1661).
Shutō shinpen	種痘新編 (*New Text on Variolation*), by Kuwata Genshin, 1814.
Shutō shinpō	種痘新法 (*A New Way to Implant Smallpox*), 1778.
Shutō hitsu jun ben	種痘必順弁 (*The Need for Inoculation*), Ogata Shunsaku, c. 1793.
Taisei meii ikō	泰西名醫彙講 (*Journal of Articles by Western Physicians*), edited by Mitsukuri Genpo, 1836–1843.
Tekijuku	適塾 The private academy founded by Ogata Kōan in Osaka; also called Tekitekisai-juku.
Tenmondai	天文台 The Astronomy Bureau of the Tokugawa government, founded in Edo by Shogun Tokugawa Yoshimune.
tenmonkata	Employees of the Tokugawa government at the Tenmondai.

tennentō	Smallpox (Japanese); *hōsō* and *tōsō* are also Japanese terms for smallpox.
"Tōka shussei"	痘科集成 (*A Manuscript on Smallpox*), by Satō Taizen.
Tokugawa	The family name of the military rulers of Japan, 1600–1867.
"Tonka hiketsu"	遁花秘訣 ("The Way to Prevent Smallpox"), translation of a Russian vaccination tract by Baba Sajūrō.
Variola major/minor	人痘苗 (*jintō byō*) The smallpox virus.
Variolae vaccinae	牛痘苗 (*gyūtō byō*) The cowpox virus.
VOC	Verenigde Oost-Indische Compagnie (Dutch East India Company).
Wada-juku	和田塾 Satō Taizen's private academy in Edo. The headship passed to Hayashi Dōkai in 1843.
yakukan	A government official.
Yakken	訳健 (*A Key to Translation*), by Fujibayashi Fusan, 1810.
yashiki	A residence, mansion.
Yi zong jin jian	医宗金艦 (*The Official Compilation: the Golden Mirror of Medicine*), Chinese book, compiled by Wu Qian, 1742.
Yin dou lue	印痘新法 (*Outline on Guiding Smallpox*), Chinese book, by Qui Xi, 1817.

Notes

NOTES FOR CHAPTER I

1. The scholarly and popular literature on the history of smallpox is enormous. It exists in many languages and spans many centuries. A short selection of historical approaches to this subject includes F. Fenner, et al. *Smallpox and Its Eradication*, History of International Public Health, No. 6 (Geneva: World Health Organization, 1988); Donald R. Hopkins, *Princes and Peasants: Smallpox in History* (Chicago: University of Chicago Press, 1983); Peter Sköld, *The Two Faces of Smallpox: A Disease and Its Prevention in Eighteenth- and Nineteenth-Century Sweden* (Umeå, Sweden: Umeå University, 1996); and J. R. Smith, *The Speckled Monster: Smallpox in England, 1670–1970* (Chelmsford, UK: Essex Record Office, 1987).

2. Genevieve Miller, *The Adoption of Inoculation for Smallpox in England and France* (Philadelphia: University of Pennsylvania Press, 1957), 27–31.

3. Ibid., 26.

4. Sköld, 229–230; Fenner, 245–257; Miller, 42–44.

5. India and Africa developed similar variolation techniques, possibly even earlier than China or Turkey, but knowledge of these techniques was disseminated less broadly to the global community.

6. A detailed history of smallpox and Chinese ideas about techniques to control it can be found in Chia-feng Chang, "Aspects of Smallpox and Its Significance in Chinese History" (Ph.D. Dissertation, University of London, 1996).

7. Chia-feng Chang, "Disease and Its Impact on Politics, Diplomacy, and the Military: The Case of Smallpox and the Manchus (1613–1795)," *Journal of the History of Medicine and Allied Sciences* 57, no. 2 (2002):182–183.

8. Ibid., 186–188.

9. Shi-yung Liu, "The Chinese Fever School in Japan" (paper presented at the MAR–AAS Annual Meeting, Pittsburgh, PA, October 1994).

10. Ibid., 8–9.

11. Harmut O. Rotermund, *Hōsōgami ou la petite vérole aisément: matériaux pour l'étude des épidémies dans le Japan des XVIIIe, XIXe siècles* (Paris: Maisonneuve & Larose, 1991), 39–45.

12. Marta E. Hanson, "The Significance of Manchu Medical Sources in the Qing." *Proceedings of the First North American Conference on Manchu Studies* (Portland, OR, May 9–10, 2003): 131–175. *Tunguso Sobirica* 15, Vol. 1: Studies in Manchu Literature and History, ed. Wadley Stephen and Carsten Naeher in collaboration with Keith Dede (Weisbaden: Harrassowitz Verlag, 2006).

13. Cited in Miller, 48.

14. Ibid.

15. It is not clear whether Chinese-style variolation's westward trek across Central Asia had an influence on Turkish-style variolation. While either technique could have influenced the other, it is equally possible that they developed independently of one another.

16. For additional references to early information about the Chinese method received by members of the Royal Society, see Miller, 48–49.

17. Ibid., 55–64.

18. Ibid., 68–69

19. Ibid., 69.

20. Ibid., 74.

21. Ibid., 82–85.

22. Ibid., 96–97. Chapters 2 and 3 in Smith provide an excellent history of inoculation in Britain.

23. Miller, 53–54.

24. Ibid., 45.

25. Lorenz Heister, *Chirurgie*, 1st ed. (Nurnberg: Johann Hoffmanns, 1719).

26. From an English translation of Heister's *Chirurgie: A General System of Surgery, in Three Parts*, 4th ed. (London: W. Innis, 1750), v–vii.

27. Ibid., vii.

28. Ibid., viii.

29. Ibid., 306–307.

30. *Nihongi: Chronicles of Japan from the Earliest Times to A.D. 697*, trans. W. G. Aston, vol. 2 (London: George Allen and Unwin, Ltd., 1956), 102–104.

31. For descriptions of smallpox in premodern Japan, see Ann Bowman Jannetta, *Epidemics and Mortality in Early Modern Japan* (Princeton, NJ: Princeton University Press, 1987), 61–107; and William Wayne Farris, *Population, Disease, and Land in Early Japan, 645–900* (Cambridge, MA: Harvard University Press, 1985), 53–69.

32. Jannetta, 67–70.

33. Cynthia Viallé and Leonard Blussé, eds., *The Deshima Dagregisters: 1641–1650*, vol. 11 (Leiden: Institute for the History of European Expansion, 2001). Intercontienta Series, No. 23, 102.

34. Jannetta, 76–97.

35. *Machi bugyō* were city administrators who governed the shogunal cities of Edo, Osaka, Kyoto, and Nagasaki, for the Tokugawa *bakufu*. They were the highest ranking officials in these cities. Two *machi bugyō* were appointed to govern Nagasaki; one lived in Edo, the other in Nagasaki, and they exchanged residences every year.

In English publications they are often called "magistrates" or "commissioners." The Dutch referred to them as "Governors."

36. Ninomiya Rikuo, *Tennentō ni idomu* (*Challenging Smallpox*) (Tokyo: Hirakawa Shuppan Sha, 1997), 186–188.

37. The editor and compiler of this work was Wu Qian. See Chang, 1996, 138, 203.

38. Ibid., 138, n. 70.

39. Soekawa Masao, *Nihon tōbyō shi shosetsu* (*An Outline History of Smallpox in Japan*) (Tokyo: Kindai Shuppan, 1987), 8–9.

40. *Isō kinkan* describes three other variation methods. One had a low success rate; a second was considered too dangerous. The third method used smallpox crusts in water and a small ball of cotton that had been immersed in water and inserted into the nostril. Soekawa, 9.

41. The infective agent in Chinese is called *miao*; in Japanese the same character is called *byō*.

42. The official rank of A. L. (Ambrosius Lodovicus) Bernardus Keller at Dejima was Oppermeester (physician), in the service of the Dutch East India Company. Viallé and Blussé, vol. 10, 204.

43. Ibid., 58–59. Discussions between the Dutch and Japanese in Edo were possible because Nagasaki interpreters were always present to translate.

44. Soekawa, 40.

45. Kumamoto Masahiro, *Ogata Shunsaku* (Amagi, Fukuoka-ken: Published by the author, 1977), 6–7, 89; Soekawa, 11.

46. Ogata Shunsaku's school register lists the names of sixty-nine physicians who came from other domains to study with him. Soekawa, 9; Sakai Shizu, *Nihon no iryō shi* (*History of Medicine in Japan*) (Tokyo: Tokyo Shoseki, 1982), 368.

NOTES FOR CHAPTER 2

1. Edward Jenner, *An Inquiry into the Causes and Effects of the Variolae Vaccinae, a Disease Discovered in Some of the Western Counties of England, Particularly Gloucestershire, and Known by the Name of the Cow Pox* (London: Printed for the author by Sampson Low, 1798), iii–iv.

2. William LeFanu, *A Bibliography of Edward Jenner*, 2nd ed. (Winchester, UK: St. Paul's Bibliographies, 1985), 5.

3. W. R. LeFanu, *A Bio-bibliography of Edward Jenner, 1749–1823* (Philadelphia: J. B. Lippincott Company, 1951), 1–14.

4. Ibid., 14–16.

5. The word "immune" is used anachronistically here; the concept of immunity was not known at the time.

6. Jenner, 6–7. The early, nonscientific meaning of "virus" was "a slimy liquid, poison, or venom." At the end of the eighteenth century, the word took on a more precise meaning: "a morbid principle or poisonous substance produced in the body as

the result of some disease, especially one capable of being introduced into other persons or animals by inoculations or otherwise and of developing the same disease in them." It was in this sense that Edward Jenner was using it. The term did not have the modern meaning of "an infectious organism that is usually submicroscopic, [and] can multiply only inside certain living host cells (in many cases causing disease)," which developed only after Louis Pasteur's articulation of the germ theory of disease in the 1880s. *Oxford Dictionary Online,* 2nd ed., 1989.

7. Ibid., 10.

8. Ibid., 31.

9. LeFanu, 1951, 28.

10. Jenner, 31–32.

11. Ibid., 32.

12. Ibid., 34. The italics are Jenner's.

13. Jenner believed that the bovine disease of cowpox was transmitted to cows by people who tended horses infected with the equine disease known as "grease," and that "true" cowpox was found only where there were horses infected with this disease. He believed that cowpox was transmitted from the horse to the cow to humans, a belief he maintained until his death. This belief was vigorously attacked at the time and has been since. The relationship between horsepox and cowpox is difficult to prove one way or the other, because neither disease survives today. Derrick Baxby, in *Jenner's Smallpox Virus: The Riddle of Vaccinia Virus and Its Origin* (London: Heinemann Educational Books, 1981), 34, suggests that Jenner's assumption may have been correct.

14. Jenner, 37. Case 19.

15. Ibid., 38. Case 20.

16. Ibid., 39. Case 21.

17. Ibid., 40. Ironically, the eleven-month-old child referred to in Case 21 was Jenner's son, Robert F. Jenner, the only recipient whose vaccination did not take.

18. Ibid., 42. Case 23.

19. LeFanu, 1985, 30. As Jenner stated in his *Inquiry,* "After many fruitless attempts to give the Small-pox to those who had had the Cow-pox, it did not appear necessary, nor was it convenient to me, to inoculate the whole of those who had been the subjects of these late trials. . . ." LeFanu, 1985, 42.

20. Jenner, 43.

21. Ibid., 44.

22. Ibid., 66.

23. Ibid., 75.

24. Richard Dunning, *Some Observations on Vaccination* (London: Cadell and Davies, 1800). Reference to Dunning's published observations on vaccination is found in LeFanu, 1985, 60.

25. LeFanu, 1985, 60.

26. Reference to George Pearson's *Inquiry Concerning the History of Cowpox, Principally with a View to Supersede and Extinguish the Smallpox* is found in Robert G. Dun-

bar, "The Introduction of the Practice of Vaccination into Napoleonic France," *Bulletin of the History of Medicine* 10, no. 5 (1941): 635-650.

27. Ibid., 637.

28. Ibid.

29. Pearson and Woodville accidentally contaminated their cowpox matter with smallpox virus, causing the children they had supposedly vaccinated to contract smallpox.

30. François Colon, *Histoire de l'introduction et des progrès de la vaccine en France* (Paris: 1801). Translated and cited in Dunbar, 638.

31. "A Box of Pox," *Harvard Magazine* (May–June 2003), 84.

32. Genevieve Miller, ed., *Letters of Edward Jenner and Other Documents Concerning the Early History of Vaccination* (Baltimore: Johns Hopkins University Press, 1983), 10.

33. Ibid., 12. De Carro's letter is published in John Baron, *The Life of Edward Jenner*, vol. 1 (London: H. Colburn, 1827), 334.

34. Miller, 10

35. Ibid., xxii; also see letter from Jenner to De Carro, 12; and correspondence in Henry E. Sigerist, ed. *Letters of Jean De Carro to Alexandre Marcet, 1794–1815*, vol. 12 Supplements to the Bulletin of the History of Medicine (Baltimore: Johns Hopkins University Press, 1950).

36. Dunbar, 641.

37. Ibid.

38. Ibid., 641. La Rochefoucould-Liancourt's return to France was announced in *Le Moniteur* on November 28, 1799, and Pearson's London Vaccination Institute was founded on December 2, 1799.

39. Ibid.

40. Ibid., 641–642.

41. Ibid., 643–644.

42. Ibid., 644.

43. This discussion of Spain's contribution to the global transmission of cowpox vaccine and vaccination is based on Michael Smith's superb account of the Spanish Royal Maritime Expedition. Michael M. Smith, "The 'Real Expedición Marítima de la Vacuna' in New Spain and Guatemala," *Transactions of the American Philosophical Society*, vol. 64 (Philadelphia: American Philosophical Society, 1974).

44. Ibid., 13. Most likely Luigi (Aloysius) Careno.

45. Ibid.

46. Ibid., 12.

47. Ibid.

48. Ibid., 14.

49. Ibid., 13. King Carlos IV encouraged variolation after his daughter was stricken with smallpox in 1798. His two sons, Carlos and Ferdinand, were variolated by the royal physicians.

50. Ibid., 17.

51. Ibid., 20.

52. Ibid.

53. Ibid., 56.

54. Ibid.

55. Ibid., 58.

56. Ibid., 59.

57. Ibid.

58. Joseph Needham and Lu Gwei-djen, "Biology and Biological Technology," in *Science and Civilisation in China,* ed. Nathan Sivin (Cambridge: Cambridge University Press, 2000), 153.

59. Smith, 59.

60. Ibid., 61.

61. Mauritius, an island in the Indian Ocean, was discovered by the Portuguese in 1505. It was occupied by the Dutch from 1598 to 1711; it was held by the French from 1715 to 1810 and renamed Île de France. The island was seized by the British in 1811 and returned to the Dutch in 1816. *Webster's New Geographical Dictionary* (Springfield, MA: Merriam-Webster Inc., 1984), 743.

62. "Batavian Republic." 2005 *Encyclopaedia Britannica Online,* January 18, 2005. http://search.eb.com/eb/article?tocId=9013717.

63. M. Laborde, "An Account of the Introduction of the Vaccine Disease into the Isles of France and Réunion," *Philadelphia Medical and Physical Journal* 11 (1805): 71–77.

64. Ibid., 71–73.

65. Confluent smallpox was an especially serious form of the disease and was almost always fatal.

66. Laborde, 73–74.

67. Ibid., 74–75.

68. This information indicates that Laborde obtained cowpox matter sometime before the end of 1803, and the French authorities were already attempting to send it to the Dutch at Batavia.

69. D. Schoute, *Occidental Therapeutics in the Netherlands East Indies During Three Centuries of Netherlands Settlement, 1600–1900* (Batavia: Publications of the Netherlands Indies Public Health Service, 1937), 96.

70. Miller, 19.

71. Ibid., 31. This letter is dated November 21, 1806. Jenner may be referring to the report in the *Gaceta de Madrid,* October 14, 1806, which describes the successful outcome of the Balmis expedition.

72. This remark, attributed to Jenner, is found in K. C. Wong and L. T. Wu, *History of Chinese Medicine: Being a Chronicle of Medical Happenings in China from Ancient Times to the Present Period* (Tientsin, China: Tientsin Press, Ltd., 1932), 143.

NOTES FOR CHAPTER 3

1. *Yōgaku shi jiten (Dictionary of the History of Western Studies)* (Tokyo: Yūshōdō Shuppan, 1984), 55–59.

2. Despite severe punishments for the Japanese who were caught dealing in contraband goods, the smuggling of goods in and out of Japan was extensive. For detailed information about smuggling and the general handling of Dutch goods that came to Nagasaki, see Martha Chaiklin, *Cultural Commerce and Dutch Commercial Culture: The Influence of European Material Culture on Japan, 1700–1850* (Leiden: Research School of Asian, African and Amerindian Studies, 2003), 21–28.

3. Cynthia Viallé and Leonard Blussé, eds. *The Deshima Dagregisters: Their Original Tables of Contents, 1790–1800,* vol. 10. Intercontinenta Series, Leiden: Institute for the History of European Expansion, 1997, i.

4. Ibid., ii.

5. Ibid.

6. Ibid.

7. Hendrik Doeff, *Herinneringen uit Japan (Memories from Japan)* (Haarlem: François Bohn, 1833), 76.

8. Baba Sajūrō, "Tonka hiketsu." Unpublished manuscript, 1820. Sen'an Toshimitsu, ed., *Roshia gyūtō zensho (Treatise on Russian Cowpox)* (Edo: publisher unknown, 1850).

9. The *Rebecca* sailed from Boston with an American captain, James Deal. Shunzō Sakamaki, "Japan and the United States, 1790–1853," *Transactions of the Asiatic Society of Japan,* vol. 18, Series 2 (Tokyo: Asiatic Society of Japan, 1939), 5–6.

10. *Yōgaku shi jiten,* 65. Jan Frederick Feilke served as the Dutch physician at Dejima during 1803 and part of 1804. Feilke was replaced by Hermanus Letzke during part of 1804 and 1805; he returned to Dejima in 1805 for a tour of several years.

11. The *Franklin,* an American ship out of Boston, arrived in Batavia on April 28, 1799. It left Batavia for Japan on June 17 and arrived in Nagasaki on July 18, 1799.

12. Doeff, 61–62.

13. Leopold Willem Ras, Scriba, served as acting Opperhoofd after Hemmij's death.

14. Viallé and Blussé, viii.

15. Doeff, 115.

16. Ibid., 116.

17. Ibid., 143–47. This translation and those of all other Dutch sources that follow were done by Frans-Paul van der Putten.

18. The names Doeff gave to Japanese high officials are routinely mentioned in Japanese biographies of these men.

19. Numata Jirō, *Western Learning: A Short History of the Study of Western Science in Early Modern Japan,* trans. R. C. J. Bachofner (Tokyo: Japanese Netherlands Institute, 1992), 112–116.

20. François Halma, ed. *Woordenboek der Nederduitsche en Fransche Taalen.* (Amsterdam: Wetsteins en Smith, 1729).

21. These sample entries are taken from a facsimile of the *Doeff haruma,* entitled *Oranda jiten* (Dutch Dictionary) published by Waseda University in 1974.

22. Initially, there were two copies of the *Doeff haruma.* One copy remained in

Japan when Hendrik Doeff returned to the Netherlands. The second copy, which Doeff took with him, was lost when the ship on which he was traveling sank.

23. It is not clear whether Baba Tamehachirō was Sajūrō's real brother, or if he too was adopted into the Baba family.

24. Numata, 101.

25. Ibid., 85-96. Shizuki Tadao was also called Nakano Ryūho. For detailed information about Shizuki Tadao's life and scholarship, see Annick Horiuchi, "When Science Develops Outside State Patronage: Dutch Studies in Japan at the Turn of the Nineteenth Century." *Early Science and Medicine* 8, no. 2 (2003): 157-159.

26. *Rekishō shinsho,* by Shizuki Tadao, is a partial translation, based on a Dutch translation of a Latin book by the Englishman John Keill (1671-1721). The original book is an explanation of Isaac Newton's theories on the solar system. The Latin title is *Introductiones ad veram Physicum et veram Astronomiam* (London, 1739). The Dutch title is *Inleidinge tot de Waare natuur en Sterrekunde* (Leiden, 1741). Numata, 92-93; Donald Keene, *The Japanese Discovery of Europe, 1720-1830,* rev. ed. (Stanford, CA: Stanford University Press, 1969), 76-77.

27. Shizuki Tadao used the edition compiled by Willem Sewel in Amsterdam in 1708.

28. George Alexander Lensen, *The Russian Push Toward Japan: Russo-Japanese Relations, 1697-1875* (Princeton: Princeton University Press, 1959), 140. Lensen gives a superb, detailed account of the meeting of the Russian crew and Japanese officials in 1804 and of the events that followed. Ibid., 138-176.

29. Ibid., 147.

30. Ibid., 167-172.

31. Ibid., 174-175.

32. *Yōgaku shi jiten,* 574.

33. The Tenmondai in Asakusa had been established half a century earlier by the eighth shogun, Tokugawa Yoshimune.

34. "Astronomers" is literal translation of the term *tenmonkata,* but it also refers to Tokugawa government employees who worked at the Tenmondai.

35. Takahashi Kageyasu (Sakuzaemon) is the person Hendrik Doeff referred to as Takahashi Sanpei.

36. Numata, 101.

37. Ibid., 102.

38. NFJ 2.21.54: Hendrik Doeff, April 15, 1808.

39. For an account of Daikokuya Kōdayū's experiences in Russia and his treatment when he returned to Japan, see Keene, 46-58.

40. The Russian vaccination tract was compiled by the Medical-Philanthropic Committee, Imperial Academy of Science, *Sposob izbavitsia povershenno ot ospennoi zarazy posredstvm vseobshchego privivaniia korovei ospy* (*Instructions on How to be Spared Infection of the Pox by Means of Universal Vaccination with Cowpox*) (Moscow: Synod Printing House, 1805).

41. Matsuki Akitomo, *Nakagawa Gorōji shoshi* (*A Bilbiography of Nakagawa Gorōji*) (Hirosaki: Aomori Prefecture, 1998), i-ii.

42. Adachi San'ai was probably chosen for this mission because he had translated a Russian arithmetic book that Daikokuya Kōdayū had brought back to Japan in 1793. Lensen, 248.

43. Vasilii Mikhailovich Golovnin, *Memoirs of a Captivity in Japan, During the Years 1811, 1812, and 1813, with Observations on the Country and People* (London: Henry Colburn and Co., 1824), vol. 2, 5–6.

44. Golovnin, 10.

45. Ibid., 37–38.

46. Murakami Teisuke, a resident of Ezo, was also serving as a Russian interpreter.

47. Baba, Preface, n. p.

48. Golovnin, 39.

49. Ibid.

50. Over the next eight years, the Russians made several attempts to establish friendly relations with Japan, but these were either ignored or rejected by the Japanese. Finally, in 1821, the Governor at Irkutsk ordered the cessation of attempts to establish official relations with Japan. In the future shipwrecked Japanese were to be sent to the Kurile Islands to find their own way home. Lensen, 262–262.

51. Ogata Tomio, *Nihon saikin gaku gaishi* (Kyoto: Maeda Shinkōdō, 1975), 4.

52. Baba, Preface, n.p.

53. Peter Gordon, "An Account of a Short Visit to Japan in 1818," *Indo-Chinese Gleaner* 8 (1819): 54–56.

54. Baba, Preface, n. p.

55. Ibid., n. p.

56. Ibid.

57. Baba Sajūrō's death date is not known. He was alive in the spring of 1822 to greet Opperhoofd Jan Cock Blomhoff when he arrived in Edo. Since 1822 was a cholera year in Japan, it is possible that Sajūrō died in the epidemic that summer or fall.

58. Soekawa Masao, *Nihon tōbyō shijosetsu (An Outline History of Smallpox in Japan)* (Tokyo: Kindai Shuppan, 1987), 25–29.

NOTES FOR CHAPTER 4

1. A detailed history of smallpox and vaccination in the Dutch East Indies can be found in Peter Boomgaard, "Smallpox and Vaccination in Java, 1780–1860: Medical Data as a Source for Demographic History." In *Dutch Medicine in the Malay Archipelago 1816–1942*, ed. A. M. Luyendijk-Elshout et al. (Amsterdam and Atlanta: Rodopi, 1989).

2. John Baron, *The Life of Edward Jenner* (London: H. Colburn, 1827–1838), vol. 2, 187.

3. Ibid.

4. Susan Legêne, *De bagage van Blomhoff en van Breugel (The Baggage of Blomhoff and van Breugel)* (Rotterdam: University of Rotterdam, 1998), 322.

5. Ibid., 159.

6. Ibid., 48. See René P. Bersma, *Titia: The First Western Woman in Japan* (Amsterdam: Hotei Publishing, 2002) for a chronology of events concerning Titia and the story from her point of view.

7. NJF 442/1118: Incoming letter from Council at Batavia to Blomhoff, June 18, 1821.

8. Ibid.

9. The title of the Dutch translation is *Algemeene beschouwing van de geschiedenis der koepokken en derzelven inenting als het zekerste en heilzaamste middel ter geheele uitroeijing der menschenpokken* (*A General View of the History of Cowpox and Cowpox Inoculation as the Surest and Most Beneficial Method for the Extermination of Smallpox*), Amsterdam, 1802.

10. NJF 695: Outgoing letter from Blomhoff to Council at Batavia, no date, 1821.

11. Ibid.

12. NJF 443/22: Incoming letter from Council at Batavia to Blomhoff, no date, 1822.

13. NJF 443/2: Excerpt from Council Resolution No. 22 sent to Blomhoff, 1822.

14. Legêne, 321.

15. NJF 1443/86: Miscellaneous Trade, Invoice from *Jonge Anthony*, 1822.

16. NJF 1443/83: Miscellaneous Trade, Invoice from *Jorina*, 1822.

17. NJF 443/1: August 16, 1822.

18. NJF 443/2: August 17, 1822.

19. Jan Cock Blomhoff's first court journey to Edo was in 1818. His private account of that journey has been edited by F. R. Effert, translated and published in English as *The Court Journey to the Shōgun of Japan* (Leiden: Hotei Publishing, 2000).

20. NJF 696: Outgoing letter from Blomhoff to Council at Batavia, November 25, 1822. Blomhoff's references to himself in the third person have been changed to the first person.

21. NJF 236: *Dagregister*, November 26, 1822 to November 20, 1823.

22. Ibid., entry for March 6, 1823.

23. Ibid., entry for March 7, 1823.

24. Presumably D. Davids refers to Dr. Leonardus Davids, who had translated Jenner's *Inquiry* into Dutch in 1801.

25. NJF 236: *Dagregister*, November 26, 1822 to November 20, 1823; entries for March 7, 1823, and March 10, 1823.

26. Jenner, *Inquiry*, p. 74. The italics are Jenner's.

27. Jenner's horsepox theory had been challenged by his British medical colleagues, but neither Blomhoff nor the Japanese physicians would have known that.

28. NJF 236: *Dagregister*, November 26, 1822 to November 20, 1823; entry for March 12, 1823.

29. Ibid., entry for March 18, 1823.

30. Ibid., entry for March 20, 1823.

31. NFJ 444/34: incoming letters from Batavia to Blomhoff, 1823. Italics have been added by the author (AJ).

32. Legêne, 160.

33. Ibid., 229.

34. NJF 2.21.05.37/4: Jan Cock Blomhoff, Dutch letters from various Japanese to Cock Blumhoff.

35. Legêne, 322.

36. Several earlier Dutch Factory doctors were also academically trained: Willem Ten Rijne, Dutch physician, Dejima 1675–1676); Englebert Kaempher, German physician, Dejima, 1690–1692; and Carl Peter Thunberg, Swedish physician, naturalist and botanist, Dejima, 1795–1796.

37. Von Siebold's decision to become a military doctor and enter colonial government service was not unusual at the time. Many of his fellow students at Würzburg also entered the Dutch colonial service when they finished their medical training, but von Siebold's appointment to the rank of Surgeon Major was unusual for a young man of twenty-six.

38. Lutz Walter, ed., "Philipp Franz von Siebold," in *Japan: A Cartographic Vision. European Printed Maps from the Early 16th to the 19th Century* (Munich: Prestel, 1994), 70.

39. *Catalogue de la bibliotèque, apportée au Japon par Mr. Ph. F. de Siebold* (Dejima: Imprimerie Néerlandaise, 1862), lists 760 writings von Siebold took to Japan. Divided into categories by topic, many of these writings predate his arrival in 1823.

40. Von Siebold has long been given credit for introducing vaccination to Japan, but neither Dutch nor Japanese contemporaneous sources make this claim, nor do Dutch scholars who have studied the sequence of events. The lymph von Siebold brought with him from Batavia proved ineffective when he vaccinated two children about two weeks after his arrival. Tadashi Yoshida, "Von Siebold as a Station Doctor." In *Philipp Franz von Siebold: A Contribution to the Study of the Historical Relations Between Japan and the Netherlands*, ed. Netherlands Association for Japanese Studies (Leiden: Netherlands Association for Japanese Studies, 1978), 36.

41. Ibid., 42.

42. Harmen Beukers, *The Mission of Hippocrates in Japan: The Contribution of Philipp Franz von Siebold* (Leiden: Foundation for Four Centuries of Netherlands-Japan Relations, 2000), 46.

43. Numata Jirō, *Western Learning: A Short History of the Study of Western Science in Early Modern Japan,* trans. R. C. J. Bachofner (Tokyo: Japanese Netherlands Institute, 1992), 118.

44. Ibid., 22–23. Narabayashi Chinzan published a treatise on Dutch surgery, *Kōi geka sōden (Red-Hair Surgery)* in 1706.

45. Ibid., 119–20.

46. Ibid. For an excellent account of von Siebold's approach to medical training in Japan see Beukers, 54–66.

47. For a detailed description of von Siebold's school, Narutaki, which includes the geographical range of students and provides details about the students and their relationship with the school, see Richard Rubinger, *Private Academies of Tokugawa Japan* (Princeton, NJ: Princeton University Press, 1982), 112–117.

48. Kure Shūzō, *Shiiboruto sensei: sono shōgai oyobi kōgyō (Dr. Siebold: His Life and*

Accomplishment) (Tokyo: Meicho Kankō Kai, 1979), 35–37. See Appendix 2 for the names and ages of von Siebold's students. Having studied with von Siebold became an important status symbol, so the list may be somewhat inflated.

49. Ibid.

50. Philipp Franz von Siebold, *Nippon: Archiv zur beschreibung von Japan und dessen Neben- und Schutzländern Jezo mit den südlichen Kurilen, Sachalin, Korea und den Liukiu-inseln (Nippon.. Archive for the Description of Japan and its Adjacent and Protected Territories, Yezo together with the Southern Kuriles, Korea, and the Ryukyu Islands)*, 2nd ed., 2 vols. (Würzberg Leipzig, L. Woerl, 1897).

51. The best information about the essays written by von Siebold's most famous students can be found in "Monjin ga Shiiboruto ni teikyō shitaru rango ronbun no kenkyū" ("The Dutch Language Essays Presented to von Siebold by His Students"), in *Shiiboruto no kenkyū (Research on von Siebold)*, ed. by Nichidoku Bunka Kyōkai (Japanese-German Cultural Society), (Tokyo: Iwanami Shoten, 1938).

52. Philipp Franz von Siebold with Joseph Gerhard Zuccarini, *Flora Japonica* (Leiden: Verfasser, 1835–1870).

53. Yoshida, 32.

54. Von Siebold's letter is dated October 30, 1824. NA *VOC* 2.10.01: Colonial Affairs March 22, 1825, n. 1.

55. Carl Peter Thunberg, *Flora Japonica*, (Leipzig: I. G. Muller, 1784).

56. Itō Keisuke undoubtedly made a substantial contribution to von Siebold's *Flora Japonica*. The first installments, in collaboration with J. G. Zuccarini, were published in 1835.

57. This translation is from the German edition of *Nippon* (Würzburg and Leipzig: L. Woerl, 1897), 188.

58. Ibid.

59. The date of departure in the Dutch calendar was May 18, 1826; in the Japanese calendar, it was the twelth day, fourth month, of the ninth year of the Bunsei era.

60. For a summary account of the Siebold Incident, see Conrad Totman, *Early Modern Japan* (Berkeley: University of California Press, 1993), 509–511. A more detailed account is given in Keene, 147–55.

61. Notable exceptions are the Narabayashi-*ryū*, the Casper-*ryū*, and the Thunberg-*ryū*, all of which are recognized by Japanese scholars.

62. The Dutch title was *Ontleedkundige tafelen*. The original German text, *Anatomischen tabellen*, was extremely popular and was translated into Latin, French, and Dutch as well as Japanese.

63. Takamasa Dōke. "Yōan Udagawa: A Pioneer of Early 19th Century Feudalistic Japan," *Japanese Studies in the History of Science* 12 (1973): 102.

64. Generation 1, Udagawa Genchū, 2, Gensen; 3, Genzui (Ensen); 4, Genshuku; 5, Genzui; 6, Genshin; 7, Yōan; 8, Kōsai.

65. Dōke, 102; Numata, 85. The *Haruma wage* was later known as the *Edo haruma* to distinguish it from the *Doeff haruma*, which was compiled later by Hendrik Doeff and the group of Nagasaki interpreters.

66. *Seisetsu naika sen'yo* (*Selections from Western Internal Medicine*), 18 vols., was published in 1793. This was a translation of a text by Johannes de Gorter published in 1744.

67. Dōke, 102.

68. Ibid., 104.

69. Ibid.

70. The quotation is from Dōke, 104. See also Numata, 87.

71. Noel Chomel, *Huishoudelijk woordenboek* (*Household Encyclopedia*), 8 vols. (Leiden: 1768–77).

72. Dōke, 105–06.

73. Ibid., 108–09.

74. Ibid.

75. Ibid.

76. Numata, 96.

77. Saburō Miyashita, "A Bibliography of the Dutch Medical Books Translated in Japanese," *Archives Internationales d'Histoire des Sciences* 25, no. 96 (1975): 26.

78. Dōke, 112.

79. Ibid., 113.

NOTES FOR CHAPTER 5

1. The designation of "peasant class" is problematic. It is based on the relevant information in the biographies of these men and may not be correct. A physician's apprentice might learn by observing and doing, but the formal study of medicine would have required the kind of formal book learning that would have been more difficult for peasant families to obtain. The particulars of their childhood education are not known, but clearly these seven men were literate when they began to study medicine, and presumably this literacy had been acquired at home or at a local school.

2. Hoashi Banri's *Kyūritsū*, a treatise on Western chemistry and physics, is based on the works of several European scientists. Details of his life and writings can be found in *Sanbyaku han kashin jinmei jiten* (*Dictionary of the Names of Retainers from Three Hundred Domains*), vol. 7 (Tokyo: Dai Nihon Insatsu, 1989), 286. See also Saburō Miyashita, "A Bibliography of the Dutch Medical Books Translated into Japanese," *Archives Internationales d'Histoire des Sciences* 25, no. 96 (1975): 11.

3. The *Edo haruma* (*Edo Halma*) had been compiled in the 1790s, but it was not available in other parts of Japan. It was also known as the *Haruma wage*.

4. *Yōgaku shi jiten* (*Dictionary of the History of Western Studies*) (Tokyo: Yūshōdō Shuppan, 1984), 599.

5. Nakano Misao, "Hino Teisai sensei" ("Dr. Hino Teisai"), *Kyoto-fu ishi kaihō* (*Bulletin of Kyoto Physicians*) 3 (1950): 3–6.

6. *Yōgaku shi jiten*, 59. Itō Sakae, *Itō Genboku den* (*A Biography of Itō Genboku*) (Tokyo: Yashio Shoten, 1978). Itō Sakae's detailed chronology of his illustrious ancestor's life is a regularly cited source for important events that concerned *ranpō* physicians in

the early nineteenth century. Annotations include excerpts from letters and official documents.

7. One of these scholars was Ōba Sessai (1805–1873), a young samurai who was also from Saga domain. Ōba Sessai, like Itō Genboku, would study under Philipp Franz von Siebold in the 1820s. *Yōgaku shi jiten*, 112–13.

8. Ibid., 325.

9. Ibid., 59. Itō, 12–13

10. Itō, 19. Some Japanese scholars question Itō Sakae's claim that Itō Genboku was part of Philipp Franz von Siebold's court journey in 1826, because Inomata Denjiemon is not listed among the official interpreters that year.

11. Ibid.

12. Ibid.

13. Ibid., 20–23.

14. Ibid., 22.

15. Aochi Rinsō, a student of Baba Sajūrō, was appointed to his teacher's position at the Tenmondai when the latter died suddenly in 1822. *Yōgaku shi jiten*, 28.

16. Rubinger's excellent chapter on private medical academies in Tokugawa Japan gives detailed information about the management of Shōsendō and the composition of the students who studied at the school. Richard Rubinger, *Private Academies of Tokugawa Japan* (Princeton, NJ: Princeton University Press, 1982), 101–125.

17. The most prominent *rangaku* scholars from Sendai domain were Otsuki Gentaku, Minato Chōan, Takano Chōei, and Ishikawa Ōsho.

18. Aoki Daisuke, *Ōtsuki Shunsai den (A Biography of Ōtsuki Shunsai)* (Sendai: Private printing, 1946) is the most important biography of Ōtsuki Shunsai, and the account here relies on this work. There is some disagreement about Ōtsuki Shunsai's year of birth, and some sources give his birth year as 1806. The year 1804 is used here to plot his career trajectory, because that is the year more commonly cited.

19. Aoki, 3.

20 Numata Jirō, *Western Learning: A Short History of Western Science in Early Modern Japan,* trans.. R. C. J. Bachofner (Tokyo: Japanese Netherlands Institute, 1992), 118.

21. *Yōgaku shi jiten*, 33; Takeoka Tomozō, *Ika jinmei jisho (Dictionary of Japanese Physician's Names)* (Kyoto: Nankōdō, 1931), 433–34.

22. The titles and a brief description of Ōtsuki Shunsai's translations are listed in Saburō Miyashita, "A Bibliography of the Dutch Medical Books Translated into Japanese," *Archives Internationales d'Histoire des Sciences* 25, no. 96 (1975), 49, 57–58. Entry numbers for these translations are 346, 429, 433, and 444.

23. Shitaya is near Tokyo's Ueno Park.

24. Ogawa Teizō, *Satō Taizen den (A Biography of Satō Taizen)* Tokyo: Juntendō Shi Hensan Iinkai, 1972. Ogawa Teizō is Satō Taizen's principal biographer. *Juntendō shi nenpyō (A Chronological Table of Juntendō University)* ed. Juntendō Hensan Iinkai (Tokyo: Juntendō Hensan Iinkai, 1974) provides a detailed chronology of Satō Taizen's life. The information here is based primarily on these sources.

25. Matsumoto Jun was formally adopted by Matsumoto Ryōho in 1849.

26. Taizen was translating the writings of C. W. Hufeland and M. J. von Chelius during this period. Ogawa, 85–89.

27. Satō Taizen and others are reputed to have studied medicine with Johannes von Niemann, but Niemann was the Opperhoofd of the Dutch Factory and had no medical background. Ogawa, 20–21.

28. *Juntendō shi nenpyō*, 5.

29. Taizen may also have left Edo for political reasons. His father, Tōsuke, had submitted a petition to the *bakufu* protesting the removal of a *daimyō* from his domain in Dewa, and this petition was under review, whereas Sakura domain was not under the direct control of the *bakufu*.

30. *Juntendō shi nenpyō*, 3.

31. Ogawa, 66–71.

32. The names of prominent physicians who studied medicine and surgery at Juntendō, and the dates when new surgical procedures were performed in the late Edo period, can be found in *Juntendō shi nenpyō*, 6–14.

33. Selected biographers of Ogata Kōan are Ogata Tomio, *Ogata Kōan den* (*A Biography of Ogata Kōan*) (Tokyo: Iwanami Shoten, 1977); Umetani Noboru, *Kōan, Tekijuku no Kenkyū* (*Research on Kōan and Tekijuku*) (Kyoto: Shibunkaku Shuppan, 1993); and Ishida Sumio, *Ogata Kōan no Rangaku* (*Ogata Kōan and Dutch Studies*), (Kyoto: Shibunkaku Shuppan, 1992). The information provided here is taken mainly from these sources.

34. Umetani, 7, 16.

35. Ogata, 55.

36. Fujino Tsunesaburō, compiler. *Ogata Kōan to Tekijuku*. (Suita-shi: Tekijuku kinenkai 1993), 17.

37. Numata, 91.

38. Ibid.

39. One of these changes was made in deference to his domain lord. In 1832, when the Lord of Ashimori named his firstborn Sannojō, Kōan was still using the name Ogata Sanpei. Claiming that it would be disrespectful to continue to use the same character for san, in his own name, Kōan changed his name again. His concern suggests a continuing sensitivity to samurai protocol, despite the fact that he had given up his samurai rank.

40. Udagawa Genshin died on Tenpō 5.12.4 (1/2/1835); Ogata Kōan left Edo for Ashimori on Tenpō 6.2.20 (3/19/1835).

41. Naka Ten'yū died Tenpō 6.3.26 (4/23/1835); Ogata Kōan left Ashimori for Osaka on Tenpō 6.4.20 (5/20/1835).

42. For the geographical distribution of students registered at Tekijuku, see Rubinger, Figure 12, 144.

43. Nagayo Sensai, *Shōkō shishi* (*An Autobiography*). In *Matsuomoto Ryōjun and Nagayo Sensai,* ed. Teizō Ogawa and Shizu Sakai (Tokyo: Heibonsha, 1980).

44. Kuwata Ryūsai's biographer is Kuwata Tadachika. *Aru ranpō-i no shōgai* (*Introduction to a Ranpō Physician*) (Tokyo: Chūō Kōronsha, 1982).

45. The Kasahara archive in Fukui City holds the writings and memorabilia of Kasahara Hakuō. The role he played in the vaccination network is examined by Ban Isoshirō, "Kasahara Hakuō no shutō fukyū katsudō," ("Kasahara Hakuō and the Transmission of Vaccination"), part 1, in *Jitsugaku shi kenkyūkai ron* (*Research on the History of Practical Science*).

46. This purge by the *bakufu* is known as the *bansha no goku*. It resulted in the arrests of two well-known *ranpō* physicians, Takano Chōei (1805–1850) and Koseki San'ei (1787–1839), and led to their imprisonment and death.

47. *Yōgaku shi jiten*, 72–76, 345, 467–68.

48. Rubinger, Chapters 4 and 5.

49. Harmen Beukers mentions Richerand, Rosenstein, Consbruch, and Tittman as authors whose works von Siebold introduced to his students. These physicians were writers of concise, popular handbooks that were useful to general practitioners of medicine in Japan. Harmen Beukers, *The Mission of Hippocrates in Japan: The Contribution of Philipp Franz von Siebold* (Leiden: Foundation for Four Centuries of Netherlands-Japan Relations, 2000), 56–58.

50. Miyashita, 62–65.

51. Table 5.2 provides only a glimpse of the many translations done by *ranpō* physicians between 1830 and 1860. See Miyashita for a bibliography of the more than 400 extant Japanese translations of Dutch-language medical texts from the late Tokugawa period.

52. Christoph Wilhelm Hufeland, *Enchiridion medicum, oder anleitung zur medizinischen praxis* (*A Guide to Medical Practice, Based on 50 Years of Medical Experience*) (Berlin: Jonas, 1836).

53. Miyashita, 36–37.

54. The title of the Dutch edition is *Enchiridion medicum. Handleiding tot de geneeskundige praktijk. Erfmaking van eeen 50-jarige ondervinding*, 2nd ed., trans. H. H. Hageman (Amsterdam, 1838).

55. Nakamura Akira, "Ogata Kōan's Hu-shi keiken ikun honyaku katei no kentō," ("An Investigation into Ogata Kōan's Translation Method"). In *Nihon ishigaku zasshi* 35 (1989): 229–260.

56. Georg Friedrich Most, *Encyklopädie der gesammten medicinischen und chirurgischen praxis* (*Encyclopedia of Medical and Surgical Practice*), 2 vols. (Leipzig: F. A. Brockhaus, 1833). The Dutch translation was published in Amsterdam, 1835–1839.

57. More than 6,500 old Dutch books were found in Japan after World War II, and the total number imported must have been much greater.

58. Mitsukuri Genpo, ed., *Taisei meii iko* (*Journal of Articles by Western Physicians*) (Edo: Suharaya Ihachi, 1836–1843). These volumes are owned by Nagasaki University.

59. Anthonij Moll and Cornelis van Eldik, eds., *Practisch tijdschrift voor de geneeskunde* (*Journal of Practical Medicine*) (Gorinchem: Jacobus Noorduyn, 1822–1856). The Japanese translations were of articles published in vol. 10 (1831) and vol. 25 (1837).

60. *Yōgaku shi jiten*, 421; Miyashita, 58.

61. Beukers, 88–90. Beukers compares the study of *materia medica* in Japan and Europe. The fact that some plants were indigenous to both places and others were not accounts for the interest of the Dutch Factory physicians who wished to look for herbal plants in the environs of Nagasaki. Some common European *materia medica*, such as belladonna and digitalis, were not indigenous to Japan.

62. Nishimura Shigeki, *Shutō no hanashi*, cited in Ogawa, 81.

63. Matsumoto Ryōjun was Satō Taizen's fourth child, second son, born in 1832.

64. Ogawa, 80.

65. Ibid., 85–89.

66. Ōtsuki Gentaku's translation of Chapter 15 on "Variolation" in Heister's *Chirurgerie* was from the 2nd Dutch edition, published in Amsterdam in 1755; Miyashita, 44.

67. Itō, 82–86.

68. Soekawa Masao, *Nihon tōbyō shi josetsu* (Tokyo: Kindai Shuppan, 1987), 183.

69. J. G. Sleeswijk, "Feuilleton: Christian Wilhelm Hufeland" in *Nederlandsch Tijdschrift voor Geneeskunde, tevens Orgaan der Nederlandsche Maatschappij tot Bevordering der Geneeskunst* (*Dutch Journal of Medical Science, also Journal of the Dutch Society for the Improvement of Medical Science*), 54, 1a (2nd series, no. 46), Amsterdam, 1910: 526–527.

70. Hufeland, *Enchiridion Medicum: or The Practice of Medicine, The Result of Fifty Years' Experience*, trans. Caspar Bruchhausen, M.S. 4th ed. (New York: William. Radde, 1855. Section on Vaccinella, 396–98).

71. Ibid.

72. NFJ 1718: Trade Report for 1843, items to be delivered in 1844: "List of books demanded by Japanese officials, 1844–1848." Masayoshi's request is listed among requests for books from the Emperor, the First Chancellor (Mizuno Echizen no Kami), and Hotta Bitchu no Kami. Requests for 1844 would have been submitted to the Dutch Factory in 1843 for shipment from Batavia the following year.

73. *Yōgaku shi jiten*, 59. Itō Genboku became personal physician to the Nabeshima family in Edo in 1844.

74. Ban, 15; and *Yōgaku shi jiten*, 674–675.

NOTES FOR CHAPTER 6

1. Sakai Shizu. *Nihon no iryō shi* (Tokyo: Tokyo Shoseki 1982), 579.

2. NJF 1618: *Dagregister*, entry for August 14, 1849.

3. The interpreters' children were Suenaga Eisuke and Nishi Keijirō. Soekawa Masao, *Nihon tōbyō shi josetsu* (*An Outline History of Smallpox in Japan*) (Tokyo: Kindai Shuppan, 1987), 45.

4. 1618 *Dagregister*, 1849. Opperhoofd Levysshon's entry for August 25, 1849.

5. Otto Mohnike, "Aanteekeningen over den Geneeskunde der Japanezen" ("Notes on the Medical Science of the Japanese"), *Vereeniging tot Bevordering der Geneeskundige Wetenschappen in Nederlandsch Indie* 1 (1853): 227.

6. NJF 1632/36: Mohnike to Levyssohn, August 31, 1849.

7. NJF 1649/29: Levysshon to the Governor of Nagasaki, September 1, 1849.

8. Nabeshima Naomasa, Lord of Saga domain, took this name in Meiji 1 (1868). In 1849 he used the name Nabeshima Kansō. *Yōgaku shi jiten* (*Dictionary of the History of Western Studies*) (Tokyo: Yūshōdō Shuppan, 1984), 526.

9. The *kokushu* included seventeen *tōzama* and three *kamon daimyō* lineages. The *tōzama daimyō* had fought against the Tokugawa at the Battle of Sekigahara in 1600. *Kamon daimyō* were related to the Tokugawa house. Conrad Totman, *Early Modern Japan* (Berkeley: University of California Press, 1993).

10. Toshio G. Tsukahira, *Feudal Control in Tokugawa Japan: The Sankin Kōtai System*, Harvard East Asian monographs, 20 (Cambridge, MA: East Asian Research Center, Harvard University Press, 1970), 25.

11. *Yōgaku shi jiten*, 526.

12. Soekawa, 45.

13. *Tennentō no zero e no michi* (*The Road to the Eradication of Smallpox*) (Tokyo: Naitō Kinen Kusuri Hakubutsukan, 1983), 106.

14. Ibid., 34. I am indebted to Kimura Sentarō, M.D., Director of Nakagawa Hospital in Fukuoka, who took me to see this striking painting at Saga City Hospital in 1998. The painting was done by Jinnouchi Shōrei in 1927. It has been moved to Saga-jō, the Saga Castle Museum, in Saga City, and a large facsimile of the painting is now on permanent display.

15. Accounts of variolation and vaccination in Japan often mention that younger daughters and younger sons were inoculated first; then, if all went well, the son and heir would be inoculated.

16. Soekawa, 33–34.

17. *Yōgaku shi jiten*, 565; *Sanbyaku han kashin jinmei jiten* (*Dictionary of Retainer Names for 300 Domains*), vol. 7 (Tokyo: Dai Nihon Insatsu, 1989), 309.

18. NJF 1632/36: Mohnike to Levyssohn, November 11, 1849.

19. Kasahara Hakuō's diary says Ka'ei 2.10.5 (November 19, 1849).

20. *Tennentō no zero e no michi*, 38.

21. Ibid.; *Yōgaku shi jiten*, 530.

22. *Tennentō no zero e no michi*, 38, 40.

23. The names of more than twenty-five physicians who participated in the distribution of cowpox vaccine in the Osaka-Kyoto region are listed. Ibid., 36.

24. From Ka'ei 2.9.15 to Ka'ei 6. Kasahara Hakuō's many writings on vaccination have been collected and preserved in the Kasahara Hakuō Collection at the Fukui Shiritsu Kyōdo Hakubutsukan (Fukui Municipal Museum). Only one of these, *Gyūtō mondō* (*Questions and Answers About Cowpox*), was published at the time. In 1989, *Senkyō roku*, Hakuō's account of the transmission of cowpox lymph from Kyoto to Fukui, was published in modern Japanese by the Fukui Municipal Museum.

25. Tsukahira, 169. The absence of the *kokushu daimyō* from Nagasaki was timed for the winter months when reverse tradewinds prevented most ships from coming to Japan from the southwest.

26. Shunsai had requested cowpox lymph from a physician in Nagoya, where

lymph was sent directly from Nagasaki by sea; however, cowpox lymph reached Edo before it arrived in Nagoya. *Tennentō no zero e no michi*, 39.

27. Ibid. The vaccination of Nabeshima Mitsuhime may have been Genboku's first vaccination and the first vaccination in Edo, but it seems more likely that the vaccination of Naomasa's daughter followed experimental trials that were not publicly acknowledged.

28. Those in attendance were Sano Jūsen, Mizumachi Bō, Maki Shundō, and others. Itō Sakae, *Itō Genboku den* (*A Biography of Itō Genboku*) (Tokyo: Genbunsha, 1916; reprint, Yashio Shoten, 1990), 89.

29. From the diary of Watanabe Yaichibei, *Watanabe Yaichibei jiseki*, cited in Ogawa Teizō, *Satō Taizen den* (*A Biography of Satō Taizen*) (Tokyo: Juntendō shi Hensan iinkai, 1972), 83.

30. Ibid., 83–84.

31. Ibid., 84.

32. *Tennentō no zero e no michi,* 36.

33. Western calendar dates are those recorded in the Dutch sources. The Dutch sources document when the *Stad Dordrecht* arrived in Nagasaki, when the first vaccinations in Nagasaki were performed, and when certain events in which the Dutch participated took place. Japanese sources can sometimes be used to confirm these dates, but Japanese calendar dates must be used to establish the timing of any events that took place after the vaccine moved to locations beyond Nagasaki.

34. The Gregorian calendar was adopted in the Netherlands in 1582.

35. For a description of how this worked in practice, see Soekawa, 59–64.

36. "Tonka hiketsu" also circulated under another title, "Orosukoku kansen tonka hiketsu" ("The Official Russian Tonka hiketsu"), which may account for Toshimitsu Sen'an's choice of title. Saburō Miyashita, "A Bibliography of the Dutch Medical Books Translated into Japanese," *Archives Internationales D'Histoire des Sciences* 25, no. 96 (1975), 53.

37. Toshimitsu Sen'an's edited version of Baba Sajūrō's "Tonka hiketsu," *Roshia gyūtō zensho*, was first published in 1850 and reprinted in 1855.

38. Other members of the vaccination network wrote in anticipation of the eventual arrival of cowpox vaccine. For example, Arima Setsuzō's translation of Goldschmidt's 1802 book on Jenner's cowpox method was completed before his death in 1847 but not published until 1849. Other translations that were never published may have circulated privately.

39. The Dutch title of Goldschmidt's original book, published in Germany in 1801, is *Algemeene beschouwing van de geschiedenis der koepokken en derzelven inenting als het zekerste en heilzaamste middel ter geheele uitroeijing der menschenpokken* (*A General View on the History of Cowpox and Cowpox Inoculation as the Surest and Most Beneficial Method for the Extermination of Smallpox*), Amsterdam, 1802.

40. Hirose Genkyō, *Shintei gyūtō kihō* (*A Newly Revised Edition of the Cowpox Method*), 1850.

41. I am indebted to Professor Shizu Sakai, Juntendō University, for alerting me

to the importance of the timing of the publication of Narabayashi Sōken's book on vaccination and its wide circulation in Japan.

42. Kuwata Ryūsai, *Intō yō ryakkai* (*A Short Commentary on Vaccination*), Edo: 1849.

43. Soekawa Masao, "Gyūtō shutō hō shorei no hanga ni tsuite" ("Woodblock Prints to Promote Cowpox Vaccination"), *Nihon Ishigaku Zasshi* (*Journal of Japanese Medical History*) 30 (1984): 64.

44. Ibid., 68–69.

45. Ibid.

46. This was a legitimate claim. Vaccination was classified as a surgical technique in nineteenth-century Europe, where information on vaccination is found in the sections on surgery in European medical textbooks.

47. Mohnike, 228–229.

NOTES FOR CHAPTER 7

1. Tsujimoto Shōan died on Ansei 4.3.6 (March 31, 1857) and Taki Motokata on Ansei 4.4.14 (May 7, 1857).

2. Brett L. Walker, "The Early Modern Japanese State and Ainu Vaccination: Redefining the Body Politic, 1799–1868," *Past and Present* 163 (May 1999): 121–160. This excellent article includes a detailed account of the Ezo vaccination campaign of 1857.

3. Abe Masahiro was a member of the "open country" faction, and he may have been favorably inclined toward *rangaku* objectives.

4. There are no reliable statistics on the population of Ezo, so it is not possible to determine whether this was a large or small proportion of the number of children at risk.

5. This account of the founding of the Otamagaike Clinic relies heavily on the work of Fukase Yasuaki, "Otamagaike shutōjo kaisetsu o megutte," ("A Consideration of the Otamagaike Vaccination Clinic"), part 2, *Nihon ishigaku zasshi* 26 (1980): 420–431.

6. Ibid., 421.

7. I am grateful for the assistance of Dr. Kimura Sentarō, who took me to see Itō Genboku's house and to visit the local school, where I was shown a copy of the comic book.

8. The names and native places of students listed on the register of Shōsendō, Itō Genboku's school, are found in *Yōgaku shi jiten* (*Dictionary of the History of Western Studies*) (Tokyo: Yūshōdō Shuppan, 1984), 74–76.

9. Juntendō Hensan Iinkai, ed., *Juntendō shi nenpyō* (*A Chronological Table of Juntendō University*) (Tokyo: Juntendō University, 1974), 6.

10. The names and native places of students in the student register of Tekijuku are found in *Yōgaku shi jiten*, 74–76.

11. Fukase, 425.

12. *Yōgaku shi jiten*, 119.

13. Ibid.

14. Sakai Shizu. *Nihon no iryo- shi* (*History of Medicine in Japan*) (Tokyo, Tokyo Shoseki, 1982), 400–402.

15. *Juntendō shi nenpyō,* 11.

16. Itō Sakae, *Itō Genboku den* (*A Biography of Itō Genboku*) (Tokyo: Genbunsha, 1916; reprint, Yashio Shoten, 1978), 63.

17. It is not remarkable that in this instance a *ranpō* physician was called to deal with the problem. Treating gunshot wounds was a surgical specialty and normally was attended to by Western-style physicians. One of the British diplomats survived; the other died.

18. Itō, 100.

19. J. L. C. Pompe van Meerdervoort, *Vijf jaren in Japan, 1857–1863* (*Five Years in Japan, 1857–1863*), vol. 2. (Leiden: Van den Heuvel & Van Santen, 1867), 179–180, 209–210. Pompe wrote that *daimyō* in the provinces of Echizen, Ise, Chikuzen, Nagato, Satsume, Hizen, Bungo, Higo, and Sado sent students to study with him in Nagasaki.

20. Ibid., 209.

21. Yoshio Izumi and Kazuo Isozumi, "Modern Japanese Medical History and the European Influence," *Keio Journal of Medicine,* 50 (2001): 96.

22. Pompe, 223–224.

23. According to the Japanese calendar, Emperor Kōmei died on Keiō 2.12.25; this date in the Western calendar is January 30, 1867. A Western journalist living in Japan at the time wrote about the immediate impact of the Emperor's death, giving his date of death as February 3, 1867. It may have been a few days before information of his death was released to the public. See John R. Black, *Young Japan, Yokohama and Yedo: A Narrative of the Settlement and the City,* vol. 2. New York: Baker, Pratt and Co., 1883, 36–38.

24. *Juntendō shi nenpyō,* 6.

25. Ibid., 8.

26. Ibid., 9.

27. Ibid.

28. Izumi and Isozumi, 96.

29. I am indebted to Nagayo Takeo, grandson of Nagayo Sensai and a physician in Nagoya, who gave me a personal copy of Sensai's autobiography, *Shōkō shishi,* the primary source for details about Sensai's life. Nagayo Sensai wrote *Shōkō shishi* in his early sixties, and it was published in 1902. It was edited by Ogawa Teizō and Sakai Shizu and published with Matsumoto Ryōjun's autobiography as *Matsumoto Jun Jiden to Nagayo Sensai Jiden* (Tokyo: Heibonsha, 1980). For a short essay in English, see also Ann Jannetta, "Nagayo Sensai," in *Doctors, Nurses, and Medical Practitioners: A Bio-Bibliographical Source Book,* ed. Lois N. Magner (Westport, CT: Greenwood Press, 1997), 199.

30. Nagayo Sensai's essay, "Kyū Ōmura-han shutō no hanashi" ("Inoculation in Old Ōmura Domain"), about his grandfather's experiments with variolation and vaccination is published with his autobiography in Ogawa and Sakai, 186–204.

31. Nagayo Sensai, *Shōkō shishi*, 112.

32. For the reign dates and life dates of the Tokugawa shoguns, see Conrad Totman, *Early Modern Japan* (Berkeley: University of California Press, 1993), 554.

33. Iwakura Tomomi (1825–1883), was a court noble who supported the Meiji restoration and became a minister of the Meiji state (1871–1883). In 1871, he headed a mission known as the Iwakura Mission to Europe and the United States.

34. Nagayo Sensai, *Shōkō shishi,* 133–134.

35. Ann Jannetta, "Problems of Classifying Deaths in Nineteenth-Century Japan," in *Registering Causes of Death,* Special Issue: *Journal of the History of Medicine and Allied Sciences* 54, 2 (1999): 294.

36. Geertz would spend the rest of his life in the employ of the Meiji government. He died of epidemic typhus in 1883 at the age of forty.

37. Geertz's letter cites statistics showing the number of vaccinations and revaccinations performed in Japan during the period from July 1, 1875, to December 31, 1877. This letter includes an English translation of the eight articles in the Sanitary Code that pertain to vaccination regulation.

38. *Eisei kyoku nenpo, 1877–1926* (*Annual Reports of the Central Sanitary Bureau. 1877–1926*). 28 vols. (Tokyo: Tōyō Shorin: Hatsubai Harashobō, 1992–1994).

39. Yamazaki Tasuku, *Nihon eki shi to bōeki shi* (*A History of Epidemics and Their Prevention in Japan*) (Tokyo: Kokuseidō, 1931), 361.

40. Ann Bowman Jannetta, and Samuel H. Preston, "Two Centuries of Mortality Change in Central Japan: The Evidence from a Temple Death Register," *Population Studies* 45, no. 3 (1991): 417–436.

41. Yamazaki, 374.

42. Ann Bowman Jannetta, Epidemics and Mortality in Early Modern Japan (Princeton, NJ: Princeton University Press, 1987), 117–144.

NOTES FOR CONCLUSION

1. Grant K. Goodman, *Japan and the Dutch, 1600–1853* (Richmond, UK: Curzon, 2000).

2. See the University of Tokyo websites at http://www.m.u-tokyo.ac.jp/html/ 2_history/history.html; http://www.m.u-tokyo.ac.jp/html/2_history/deans.html

References

ARCHIVAL COLLECTIONS USED

The following collections are in the National Archive in The Hague, The Netherlands:

Company Archives

NFJ: Nederlandse Factorij Japan, 1609–1860 (Dutch Factory in Japan, 1609–1860)

Family Archives

Jan Cock Blomhoff
Hendrik Doeff

WORKS CITED

"A Box of Pox," *Harvard Magazine.* May–June 2003: 84.
Asahi Nihon rekishi jinbutsu jiten (Japanese Historical Name Dictionary). Tokyo: Asahi Shinbunsha, 1994.
Ainslie, Whitelaw. "Observations Respecting the Small-Pox and Inoculation in Eastern Countries; with some Account of the Introduction of Vaccination into India." *Transactions of the Asiatic Society* 2, no. 52 (1830): 52–73.

Aoki Daisuke, Ōtsuki Shunsai den (A Biography of Ōtsuki Shunsai). Sendai: Private printing, 1946.

Baba Sajūrō. "Tonka hiketsu" ("How to Escape Smallpox"). In Toshimitsu Sen'an, ed. Roshia gyūtō zensho (Treatise on Russian Cowpox), ed. Toshimitsu Sen'an. Edo: publisher unknown, 1850.

Ban Isoshirō. "Kasahara Hakuō no shutō fukyū katsudō." (Kasahara Hakuō and the Transmission of Vaccination"). In Jitsugaku shiryō kenkyūkai ron, 1986: 151–194.

Baron, John. The Life of Edward Jenner, M.D., LL.D., F.R.S., Physician Extraordinary to the King, with Illustrations of his Doctrines and Selections from his Correspondence. 2 vols. London: H. Colburn, 1827–38.

Baxby, Derrick. Jenner's Smallpox Virus: The Riddle of Vaccinia Virus and Its Origin. London: Heinemann Educational Books, 1981.

Bersma, René P. Titia: The First Western Woman in Japan. Amsterdam: Hotei Publishing, 2002.

Beukers, Harmen. "The Fight Against Smallpox in Japan: The Value of Western Medicine Proved." In Red-Hair Medicine, Dutch-Japanese Medical Relations, ed. by H. Beukers, A. M. Luyendijk-Elshout, M. E. van Opstall, and Ken Vos. Amsterdam: Rodopi, 1991, 58–77.

————. The Mission of Hippocrates in Japan: The Contribution of Philipp Franz von Siebold. Leiden: Foundation for Four Centuries of Netherlands-Japan Relations, 2000.

Black, John R. Young Japan, Yokohama and Yedo. A Narrative of the Settlement and the City, 2 vols., vol. 2. New York: Baker, Pratt and Co., 1883.

Blomhoff, Jan Cock. The Court Journey to the Shōgun of Japan, trans. Mark Poysden, ed. F. R. Effert. Leiden: Hotei Publishing, 2000.

Boomgaard, Peter. "Smallpox and Vaccination in Java, 1780–1860: Medical Data as a Source for Demographic History." In Dutch Medicine in the Malay Archipelago 1816–1942, ed. A. M. Luyendijk-Elshout et al., 119–32. Amsterdam and Atlanta: Rodopi, 1989.

————. "Smallpox, Vaccination, and the Pax Neerlandica. Indonesia, 1550– 1930." Bijdragen, tot de Taal-, Land- en Volkenkunde 159, no. 4 (2003): 590–617.

Catalogue de la bibliotèque, apportée au Japon par Mr. Ph. F. de Siebold. Dejima: Imprimerie Néerlandaise, 1862.

Chaiklin, Martha. Cultural Commerce and Dutch Commercial Culture: The Influence of European Material Culture on Japan, 1700–1850. Leiden: Research School of Asian, African and Amerindian Studies, 2003.

Chang, Chia-feng. "Aspects of Smallpox and Its Significance in Chinese History." Ph.D. Dissertation, University of London, 1996.

————. "Disease and Its Impact on Politics, Diplomacy, and the Military: The Case of Smallpox and the Manchus (1613–1795)." Journal of the History of Medicine and Allied Sciences 57, no. 2 (2002): 177–197.

Chomel, Noel. Huishoudelijk woordenboek (Household Encyclopedia), 8 vols. Leiden: 1768–1777.

Colon, François. *Histoire de l'introduction et des progrès de la vaccine en France* (A History of the Introduction and Progress of Vaccine in France). Paris: 1801.

Doeff, Hendrik. *Herinneringen uit Japan* (Memories from Japan). Haarlem: François Bohn, 1833.

Dōke, Takamasa. "Yōan Udagawa: A Pioneer of Early 19th Century Feudalistic Japan," *Japanese Studies in the History of Science* 12 (1973): 99–120.

Dreyfus, Ferdinand. *Un Philanthrope d'Autrefois: La Rochefoucauld-Liancourt, 1747–1827* (Philanthropist from Another Time: La Rochefoucauld-Liancourt, 1747–1827). Paris, 1903.

Dunbar, Robert G. "The Introduction of the Practice of Vaccination into Napoleonic France." *Bulletin of the History of Medicine* 10, no. 5 (1941): 635–650.

Dunning, Richard. *Some Observations on Vaccination*. London: Cadell and Davies, 1800.

Eisei kyoku nenpo, 1877–1926 (Annual Reports of the Central Sanitary Bureau, 1877–1926), 28 vols. Tokyo: Tōyō Shorin: Hatsubai Harashobō, 1992–1994.

Farris, William Wayne. *Population, Disease, and Land in Early Japan, 645–900*. Cambridge, MA: Harvard University Press, 1985.

Fenner, Frank, et al. *Smallpox and Its Eradication*, History of International Public Health, No. 6. Geneva: World Health Organization, 1988.

Fujino Tsunesaburō, compiler. *Ogata Kōan to Tekijuku*. Suita-shi: Tekijuku Kinenkai, 1993.

Fukase Yasuaki. "Otamagaike shutōjo kaisetsu o megutte" (A Consideration of the Otamagaike Vaccination Clinic"), part 2, *Nihon ishigaku zasshi* 26 (1980): 420–431.

Geertz, A. J. C. "Vaccination in Japan," *Japan Weekly Mail*, Yokohama, June 12, 1879.

Golovnin, Vasilii Mikhailovich. *Memoirs of a Captivity in Japan, During the Years 1811, 1812, and 1813, with Observations on the Country and People*, 2 vols. London: Henry Colburn and Co., 1824.

Goodman, Grant K. *Japan and the Dutch, 1600–1853*. Richmond, UK: Curzon, 2000.

Gordon, Peter. "An Account of a Short Visit to Japan in 1818," *Indo-Chinese Gleaner* 8 (1819): 53–59.

Hanson, Marta E. "The Significance of Manchu Medical Sources in the Qing." *Proceedings of the First North American Conference on Manchu Studies* (Portland, OR, May 9–10, 2003): 131–175. *Tunguso Sibirica* 15, Vol. 1: *Studies in Manchu Literature and History*, ed. Wadley Stephen and Carsten Naeher in collaboration with Keith Dede. Weisbaden: Harrassowitz Verlag, 2006.

Heister, Lorenz. *Chirurgie, in welcher alles, was zur Wund-Artzney gehöret, nach der neuesten und besten Art, gründlich abgehandelt . . . werden,* 1st German ed. Nürnberg: Johann Hoffmanns, 1719.

Heister, Laurence (Lorenz). *A General System of Surgery, in Three Parts*. Translated from the Latin into English, 4th ed. London: W. Innis, 1740.

Hirose Genkyō. *Shintei gyūtō kihō* (A Newly Revised Edition of the Cowpox Method). 1850.

Hopkins, Donald R. *Princes and Peasants: Smallpox in History*. Chicago: University of Chicago Press, 1983.

Horiuchi, Annick. "When Science Develops Outside State Patronage: Dutch Studies in Japan at the Turn of the Nineteenth Century." *Early Science and Medicine* 8 (2003): 157–159.

Hufeland, Christoph Wilhelm. *Enchiridion medicum, oder anleitung zur medizinischen praxis* (*A Guide to Medical Practice, Based on 50 Years of Medical Experience*), Berlin: Jonas, 1836.

———. *Enchiridion Medicum: or The Practice of Medicine, the Result of Fifty Years Experience*. 4th edition. Translated by Caspar Bruchhausen. New York: Wm. Radde, 1855.

Ishida Sumio. *Ogata Kōan no rangaku* (Ogata Kōan and Dutch Studies). Kyoto: Shibunkaku Shuppan, 1992.

Itō Sakae. *Itō Genboku den* (*A Biography of Itō Genboku*). Tokyo: Genbunsha, 1916; reprint, Yashio Shoten, 1978.

Izumi, Yoshio, and Isozumi, Kazuo. "Modern Japanese Medical History and the European Influence." *Keio Journal of Medicine* 50 (2001): 91–99.

Jannetta, Ann. "Problems of Classifying Deaths in Nineteenth-Century Japan," in *Registering Causes of Death*, Special Issue: *Journal of the History of Medicine and Allied Sciences* 54, 2 (1999): 285–295.

———. "Public Health and the Diffusion of Vaccination in Japan." In *Asian Population History*, ed. Ts'ui-jung Liu. Oxford: Oxford University Press, 2001.

Jannetta, Ann Bowman. *Epidemics and Mortality in Early Modern Japan*. Princeton, NJ: Princeton University Press, 1987.

———. "From Physician to Bureaucrat: The Case of Nagayo Sensai." In *New Directions in the Study of Meiji Japan*, ed. by Helen Hardacre and Adam L. Kern. Leiden: E. J. Brill, 1997.

———. "Nagayo Sensai." In *Doctors, Nurses, and Medical Practioners: A Bio-Bibliographical Source Book*, ed. Lois N. Magner, 198–204. Westport, CT: Greenwood Press, 1997.

——— and Samuel H. Preston. "Two Centuries of Mortality Change in Central Japan: The Evidence from a Temple Death Register," *Population Studies* 45, no. 3 (1991): 417–436.

Jansen, Marius B. *The Making of Modern Japan*. Cambridge, MA: The Belnap Press of Harvard University, 2000.

Jenner, Edward. *An Inquiry into the Causes and Effects of the Variolae Vaccinae, a Disease Discovered in Some of the Western Counties of England, Particularly Gloucestershire, and Known by the Name of the Cow Pox*. London: Printed for the author by Sampson Low, 1798.

Juntendō Hensan Iinkai, ed. *Juntendō shi nenpyō* (*A Chronological Table of Juntendō University*). Tokyo: Juntendō University, 1974.

Kasahara Hakuō. *Gyūtō mondō* (*Questions and Answers about Cowpox*). Kyoto: Kyukyodo, 1850.

Kasahara Hakuō. *Senkyō roku.* Fukui: Fukui Shiritsu Kyōdo Rekishi Hakubutsukan, 1849–1853.

Keene, Donald. *The Japanese Discovery of Europe, 1720–1830,* rev. ed. Stanford, CA: Stanford University Press, 1969.

Kornicki, Peter F. *The Book in Japan: A Cultural History from the Beginnings to the Nineteenth Century.* Leiden and Boston: Brill, 1998.

———. "Castaways and Orientalists: the Russian Route to Japan in the Early Nineteenth Century." Paolo Beonio-Brocchieri Memorial Lectures in Japanese Studies. Venezia: Università ca' Foscari, 1999.

Kulmus, Johann Adam. *Anatomischen Tabellen.* Danzig: C. von Beughem, 1725.

Kumamoto Masahiro. *Ogata Shunsaku* (Ogata Shunsaku). Amagi, Fukuoka- ken: Published by the author, 1977.

Kure Shūzō. *Shiiboruto sensei: sono shōgai oyobi kōgyō* (*Dr. Siebold: His Life and Accomplishments*). Tokyo: Meicho Kankō Kai, 1979.

Kuwata Ryūsai. *Gyūtō Hatsumō* (*Dispelling Ignorance About Cowpox*). Edo, 1849.

———. *Intō yō ryakkai* (*A Short Commentary on Vaccination*). Edo: 1849.

Kuwata Tadachika. *Aru Ranpō-i no shōgai* (*Introduction to a Ranpō Physician*). Tokyo: Chūō Kōronsha, 1982.

Laborde, M. "An Account of the Introduction of the Vaccine Disease into the Isles of France and Réunion." *Philadelphia Medical and Physical Journal* 11 (1806): 71–77.

LeFanu, W. R. *A Bio-bibliography of Edward Jenner, 1749–1823.* Philadelphia: J. B. Lippincott Company, 1951.

LeFanu, William. *A Bibliography of Edward Jenner,* 2nd ed. Winchester, UK: St. Paul's Bibliographies, 1985.

Legêne, Susan. *De baggage van Blomhoff en van Breugel* (*The Baggage of Blomhoff and van Breugel*). Rotterdam: University of Rotterdam, 1998.

Lensen, George Alexander. *The Russian Push toward Japan: Russo-Japanese Relations, 1697–1875.* Princeton, NJ: Princeton University Press, 1959.

———. *Russia's Eastward Expansion.* Englewood Cliffs, NJ: Prentice-Hall, 1964.

Lindeboom, Gerrit Arie. *Dutch Medical Biography.* Amsterdam: Rodopi, 1984.

Liu, Shi-yung. "The Chinese Fever School in Japan." Paper presented at the MAR-AAS Annual Meeting, Pittsburgh, PA, October 1994.

Magner, Lois N., ed. *Doctors, Nurses, and Medical Practitioners: A Bio-bibliographical Sourcebook.* Westport: CT: Greenwood Press, 1997.

Matsuki Akitomo. *Nakagawa Gorōji shoshi* (*Nakagawa Gorōji Bibliography*). Hirosaki: Aomori Prefecture, private publication, 1998.

Medical-Philanthropic Committee, Imperial Academy of Science, Compiler. *Sposob izbavitsia povershenno ot ospennoi zarazy posredstvm vseobshchego provivaniia korovei ospy* (*Instructions on How to be Spared Infection of the Pox by Means of Universal Vaccination with Cowpox*). Moscow: Synod Printing House, 1805.

Miller, Genevieve. *The Adoption of Inoculation for Smallpox in England and France.* Philadelphia: University of Pennsylvania Press, 1957.

————, ed. *Letters of Edward Jenner and Other Documents Concerning the Early History of Vaccination.* Baltimore: Johns Hopkins University Press, 1983.

Mitsukuri Genpo, ed. *Taisei meii iko (Journal of Articles by Western Physicians)*, 8 vols. Edo: Suharaya Ihachi, 1836–1843.

Miyashita, Saburō. "A Bibliography of the Dutch Medical Books Translated into Japanese." *Archives Internationales d'Histoire des Sciences* 25, no. 96 (1975): 8–72.

Mohnike, Otto. "Aanteekeningen overden Geneeskunde der Japanezen" ("Notes on the Medical Science of the Japanese"), *Vereeniging tot Bevordering der Geneeskundige Wetenschappen in Nederlandsch Indie* 1 (1853): 25- 61; 198–300.

Mokyr, Joel. *The Gifts of Athena: Historical Origins of the Knowledge Economy.* Princeton, NJ: Princeton University Press, 2002.

Moll, Anthonij, and Cornelis van Eldik, eds. *Practisch tijdschrift voor de Geneeskunde (Journal of Practical Medicine)*. Gorinchem: Jacobus Noorduyn, 1822–1856.

"Monjin ga Shiiboruto ni teikyō shitaru rango ronbun no kenkyū" ("The Dutch Language Essays Presented to von Siebold by His Students"). In *Shiiboruto no kenkyū (Research on von Siebold)*, ed. Nichidoku Bunka Kyōkai (Japanese-German Cultural Society). Tokyo: Iwanami Shoten, 1938.

Most, Georg Friedrich. *Encyklopädie der gesammten medicinischen und chirurgischen praxis. (Encyclopedia of Medical and Surgical Practice)*, 2 vols. Leipzig: F. A. Brockhaus, 1833.

Murayama Shichirō. "Nihon saisho no gyūtō bunken no gensho" ("A Bibliography of Japan's Earliest Sources on Cowpox"). *Juntendō Medical Journal* 11, no. 2 (1965): 109–16.

Nagayo Sensai, "Kyū Ōmura-han shutō no hanashi" ("Inoculation in old Ōmura domain"). In *Matsumoto Jun to Nagayo Sensai*, ed. Ogawa Teizō and Sakai Shizu. Tokyo: Heibonsha, 1980.

————. *Shōkō shishi (An Autobiography)*. In *Matsumoto Ryōjun and Nagayo Sensai*, eds. Teizō Ogawa and Shizu Sakai. Tokyo: Heibonsha, 1980.

Nagayo Takeo. *History of Japanese Medicine in the Edo Era: Its Social and Cultural Backgrounds.* Nagoya, Japan: University of Nagoya Press, 1991.

Nakamura Akira. "Ogata Kōan's Hu-shi keiken ikun honyaku katei no kentō" ("An Investigation into Ogata Kōan's Translation Method"). *Nihon ishigaku zasshi* 35 (1989): 229–260.

Nakamura, Ellen Gardner. *Practical Pursuits: Takano Chōei, Takahashi Keisaku, and Western Medicine in Nineteenth-Century Japan.* Cambridge, MA: Harvard University Asian Center, 2005.

Nakano Misao. "Hino Teisai sensei" ("Dr. Hino Teisai"). *Kyoto fu ishi kaihō* 3 (1950): 3–6.

Narabayashi Sōken. *Gyūtō shōkō (A Few Thoughts About Cowpox)*. Nagasaki, 1849.

Needham, Joseph, and Lu Gwei-djen. "Biology and Biological Technology," in *Science and Civilisation in China*, ed. Cambridge: Cambridge University Press, 2000.

Nihongi: Chronicles of Japan from the Earliest Times to A.D. 697, vol. 2, trans. W. G. Aston. London: George Allen and Unwin, 1956.

Ninomiya Rikuo. *Kuwata Ryūsai sensei* (Dr. *Kuwata Ryūsai*). Tokyo: Kuwata Ryūsai Sensei Kenshōkai, 1998.

————. *Tennentō ni idomu* (*Challenging smallpox*). Tokyo: Hirakawa Shuppansha, 1997.

Numata, Jirō. *Western Learning: A Short History of the Study of Western Science in Early Modern Japan*. Trans. R. C. J. Bachofner. Tokyo: Japanese Netherlands Institute, 1992.

Ogata Kōan. *Ogata Kōan no tegami* (*Letters of Ogata Kōan*), ed. Ogata Tomio. Tokyo: Saine shuppan. 1980–1994.

Ogata Tomio. *Ogata Kōan den* (*A Biography of Ogata Kōan*). Tokyo: Iwanami Shoten, 1977.

Ogawa Teizō. *Satō Taizen den* (*A Biography of Satō Taizen*). Tokyo: Juntendō Shi Hensan Iinkai, 1972.

———— and Sakai Shizu, eds. *Matsumoto Jun to Nagayo Sensai* (*Matsumoto Jun and Nagayo sensai*). Tokyo: Heibonsha, 1980.

Pompe van Meerdervoort, J. L. C. *Vijf jaren in Japan, 1857–1863* (*Five Years in Japan, 1857–1863*). 2 vols. Leiden, Van den Heuvel & Van Santen, 1867–1868.

Pott, P. F. "Philipp Franz Von Siebold as a Museologist." In *Philipp Franz Von Siebold: A Contribution to the Study of the Historical Relations Between Japan and the Netherlands*. Amsterdam: Netherlands Association for Japanese Studies, 1978.

Raffles, Sir Stamford. *Report on Japan to the Secret Committee of the English East India Company*, ed. C.B.E. M. Paske-Smith. London and Dublin: Curzon Press, 1971.

"Report of Jenner's Experiments in Gloucestershire." In *Bibliotèque britannique; ou recueil extrait des ouvrages anglais périodiques, & autres sciences et arts*, October 9 (1798): 195–196.

Rotermund, Harmut O. *Hōsōgami ou la petite vérole aisément: matériaux pour l'étude des épidémies dans le Japan des XVIIIe, XIXe siècles*. (*The Smallpox God and a Light Case of Smallpox: Material for the Study of Epidemics in Japan in the 18th and 19th Centuries*). Paris: Maisonneuve & Larose, 1991.

Rubinger, Richard. *Private Academies of Tokugawa Japan*. Princeton, NJ: Princeton University Press, 1982.

Sakai Shizu. *Nihon no iryō shi* (*History of medicine in Japan*). Tokyo: Tokyo Shoseki, 1982.

Sakamaki Shunzō. "Japan and the United States, 1790–1853," *Transactions of the Asiatic Society of Japan*, vol. 18, Series 2. Tokyo: Asiatic Society of Japan, 1939.

Sanbyaku han kashin jinmei jiten (*Dictionary of Names of Retainers for 300 Domains*), 7 vols. Tokyo: Dai Nihon Insatsu, 1989.

Schoute, D. *Occidental Therapeutics in the Netherlands East Indies During Three Centuries of Netherlands Settlement, 1600–1900*. Batavia: Publications of the Netherlands Indies Public Health Service, 1937.

Siebold, Philipp Franz von. *Nippon. Archiv zur beschreibung von Japan und dessen Neben- und Schutzländern Jezo mit den südlichen Kurilen, Sachalin, Korea und den Liukiu-inseln* (*Nippon. Archive for the Description of Japan and its Adjacent and Protected Territories, Yezo together with the Southern Kuriles, Korea, and the Ryukyu Islands*), 2nd ed. 2 vols. Würzberg Leigzig: L. Woerl, 1897.

Sigerist, Henry E., ed. *Letters of Jean de Carro to Alexandre Marcet, 1794–1815,* vol. 12, Supplements to the Bulletin of the History of Medicine. Baltimore: Johns Hopkins University Press, 1950.

Sköld, Peter. *The Two Faces of Smallpox: A Disease and Its Prevention in Eighteenth- and Nineteenth-Century Sweden.* Ůmea, Sweden: Ůmea University, 1996.

Smith, J. R. *The Speckled Monster: Smallpox in England, 1670–1970, with Particular Reference to Essex.* Chelmsford, UK: Essex Record Office, 1987.

Smith, Michael M. "The 'Real Expedición Marítima de la Vacuna' in New Spain and Guatemala," *Transactions of the American Philosophical Society,* vol. 64. Philadelphia: American Philosophical Society, 1974.

Soekawa Masao. *Gyūtō shutō hō shorei no hanga ni tsuite (Woodblock Prints to Promote Cowpox Vaccination).* Nihon ishigaku zasshi 30 (1984): 62–84.

———. *Nihon tōbyō shi josetsu (An Outline History of Smallpox in Japan).* Tokyo: Kindai Shuppan, 1987.

Suda, Keizō, and Masao Soekawa. "Smallpox Mortality in a Mountainous District in Japan Where Neither Variolation nor Vaccination Had Been Performed." *Nihon ishigaku zasshi* 29 (1983): 1–12

Sugita Genpaku. *Dawn of Western Science in Japan.* Translation of *Rangaku koto hajime* by Ogata Tomio. Tokyo: Hokuseido Press, 1969.

Takeoka Tomozō. *Ika jinmei jisho (Dictionary of Physicians' Names).* Kyoto: Nankōdō, 1931.

Tennentō no zero e no michi (The Road to the Eradication of Smallpox). Tokyo: Naitō Kinen Kusuri Hakubutsukan, 1983.

Thiede, A., Y. Hiki, and G. Keil. *Philipp Franz von Siebold and His Era.* Berlin: Springer, 2000.

Tōgo, Tsukuhara. "The Founder of Western Chemistry in Japan, Udagawa Yōan." In *Bridging the Divide: 400 Years, the Netherlands–Japan,* ed. Leonard Blusse, Willem Remmelink, and Ivo Smits. Leiden: Hotei Publishers, 2000.

Toshimitsu Sen'an, ed. *Roshia gyūtō zensho (A Russian Book on Cowpox).* Edo: Publisher unknown, 1850.

Totman, Conrad. *Early Modern Japan.* Berkeley: University of California Press, 1993.

Tsukahara Tōgo, "The Founder of Western Chemistry in Japan, Udagawa Yōan" In *Bridging the divide: 400 Years, the Netherlands–Japan,* ed. Léonard Blussé, Willem Remmelink, and Ivo Smits. Leiden: Hotei Publishing, 2000.

Tsukahira, Toshio G. *Feudal Control in Tokugawa Japan: The Sankin Kōtai System.* Harvard East Asian Monographs, 20. Cambridge, MA: East Asian Research Center, Harvard University Press, 1970.

Uchida Masao, compiler. *Nihon rekjitsu genten (Dictionary of Japanese Historical Calendar).* Tokyo: Yūzankaku, 1975–1981.

Umetani Noboru. *Kōan, Tekijuku no kenkyū (Research on Ogata Kōan and Tekijuku).* Kyoto: Shibunkaku shuppan, 1993.

Viallé, Cynthia, and Leonard Blussé, eds. *The Deshima Dagregisters, 1641–1650*, vol. 11. Leiden: Institute for the History of European Expansion, 2001. Intercontinenta Series, No. 23.

———, eds. *The Deshima Dagregisters, 1790–1800. Their Original Tables of Contents*, vol. 10. Leiden: Institute for the History of European Expansion, 1997. Intercontinenta Series, No. 21.

Walker, Brett L. "The Early Modern Japanese State and Ainu Vaccinations: Redefining the Body Politic, 1799-1868." *Past and Present* 163 (May 1999): 121–160.

Walter, Lutz, ed. *Japan: A Cartographic Vision: European Printed Maps from the Early 16th to the 19th Century*. Munich: Prestel-Verlag, 1994.

Webster's New Geographical Dictionary. Springfield, MA: Merriam-Webster, 1984.

Wong, K. C., and L. T. Wu. *History of Chinese Medicine: Being a Chronicle of Medical Happenings in China from Ancient Times to the Present Period*. Tientsin, China: Tientsin Press, Ltd., 1932.

Yamazaki Tasuke. *Nihon eki shi to bōeki shi (A History of Epidemics and Their Prevention in Japan)*. Tokyo: Kokuseidō, 1931.

Yōgaku shi jiten (Dictionary of the History of Western Studies). Tokyo: Yūshōdō Shuppan, 1984.

Yoshida, Tadashi. "'Dutch Studies' and Natural Sciences." In *Bridging the Divide: 400 Years, the Netherlands–Japan*, ed. Leonard Blusse, Willem Remmelink, and Ivo Smits. Leiden: Hotei Publishers, 2000.

———. "Von Siebold as a Station Doctor." In *Phillip Franz von Siebold: A Contribution to the Study of the Historical Relations Between Japan and the Netherlands*, ed. Netherlands Association for Japanese Studies. Leiden: Netherlands Association for Japanese Studies, 1978.

Index